OSTEOPATHIC MEDICINE RECALL

Editors

Andrew D. Mosier
University College of Osteop
Doctors Hospital at Stork Co
Beachwood, Ohio

Dai Kohara
University College of Osteopathic Medicine (OUCOM)
Cuyahoga Falls General Hospital
Medina, Ohio

Wolters Kluwer | Lippincott Williams & Wilkins
Health
Philadelphia · Baltimore · New York · London
Buenos Aires · Hong Kong · Sydney · Tokyo

Acquisitions Editor: Donna Balado
Managing Editor: Cheryl W. Stringfellow
Marketing Manager: Emilie Linkins
Production Editor: Kevin P. Johnson
Designer: Teresa Mallon
Compositor: International Typesetting and Composition
Printer: R.R. Donnelley, Crawfordsville

351 West Camden Street
Baltimore, MD 21201

530 Walnut Street
Philadelphia, PA 19106

The publisher is not responsible (as a matter of product liability, negligence, or otherwise) for any injury resulting from any material contained herein. This publication contains information relating to general principles of medical care that should not be construed as specific instructions for individual patients. Manufacturers' product information and package inserts should be reviewed for current information, including contraindications, dosages, and precautions.

Printed in the United States of America

Library of Congress Cataloging-in-Publication Data

Mosier, Andrew D.
   Osteopathic medicine recall/Andrew D. Mosier, Dai Kohara.
       p. ; cm.—(Recall series)
   Includes bibliographical references and index.
   ISBN-13: 978-0-7817-6621-0
   ISBN-10: 0-7817-6621-4
   1.   Osteopathic medicine–Miscellanea.   I. Kohara, Dai.   II. Title.   III.
Series.
   [DNLM: 1. Manipulation, Osteopathic—Examination Questions.   2.
Osteopathic Medicine—Examination Questions.   WB 18.2 M911o 2007]
   RZ343.M67 2007
   615.5'33—dc22

                                     2006037180

The publishers have made every effort to trace the copyright holders for borrowed material. If they have inadvertently overlooked any, they will be pleased to make the necessary arrangements at the first opportunity.

Careful time and attention has been taken to make certain that the information contained within OMT Osteopathic Medicine Recall is correct and compatible with the standards of care accepted at the time of publication. However, the authors, editors, and publishers are not responsible for errors or omissions of information, or for any consequences from application of information in the book. Application of information from the book for any situation remains the professional responsibility of the physician. In light of ongoing research, changing government regulations upon the field of medicine, and the constant influx of information relating to the book, the reader is always urged to confer with the most updated primary sources for added knowledge, warning, and precautions.

To purchase additional copies of this book, call our customer service department at **(800) 638-3030** or fax orders to **(301) 223-2320**. International customers should call **(301) 223-2300**.

Visit Lippincott Williams & Wilkins on the Internet: http://www.LWW.com. Lippincott Williams & Wilkins customer service representatives are available from 8:30 am to 6:00 pm, EST.

07 08 09 10
1 2 3 4 5 6 7 8 9 10

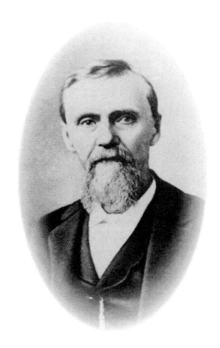

A.T. Still, the father of osteopathic medicine

Dedication

This book is dedicated to the entire dedicated faculty at Ohio University College of Osteopathic Medicine who encouraged us as students to master the fundamentals of osteopathic medicine. We would like to give special mention to Dr. Janet Burns, D.O., who spent countless hours encouraging us to follow our dreams to become knowledgeable physicians and help bring light to the field of osteopathic medicine.

We would also like to devote this book to our families: Sue, Dennis, and Cindy Mosier, Aaron and Erin, Heidi, the "Chicago" Otts, Justin, Haruki, and Kazuyo Kohara for always believing in our far-reaching goals. Without your love and support we could not have made it this far.

Preface

Osteopathic Medicine Recall presents both students and teachers with an up-to-date approach to learning and reviewing the basics of osteopathic medicine. The book uses a short question and answer format, addressing key principles and high-yield information while maintaining the concept of the Recall Series that continues to be so widely utilized by medical students and physicians throughout the world. The question and answer format gives the reader a chance to effectively review and read the most commonly tested fundamentals, setting up a dialogue in the reader's mind that will assist in mastering the information.

Osteopathic Medicine Recall is divided into 14 chapters to address topics in a logically presented fashion that will make sense to the reader. The book has a strong emphasis on basic knowledge in osteopathic medicine, for it is our belief as fellow students that there is no concept too difficult to learn if the fundamentals are properly applied. For this reason, the book begins with a quick review of the most basic concepts in osteopathic medicine. Following the first chapter is a section devoted to both the axial and appendicular spine, the core of osteopathic medicine. Beginning with Chapter 4, select high-yield information is broken down into easy-to-read chapters that the reader should find both time effective and manageable.

This book should be used by the reader as a guide to understanding more difficult osteopathic texts, studying for board examinations, and recalling forgotten information quickly before hospital and office rotations where techniques can be practically applied. The reader may choose to read through the book in short pieces between classes or while studying at night individually or with a group of colleagues. The book has also been designed so that the reader may read through the book in one weekend to brush up on the fundamentals of osteopathic medicine before a critical test. *Osteopathic Medicine Recall* was created to be a study guide with references listed for further reading. Many questions are concept questions with answers condensed from multiple paragraphs and sometimes pages. The corresponding references have been listed to give you, the reader, the page(s) that best expound upon the answer provided for each question. The list of works cited appears in the back of the book.

Please feel free to contact us if you have noted any acronyms that we may have overlooked or not used, if you have any corrections, or if you have any suggestions for possible future editions. You can reach us by e-mail in care of Lippincott Williams & Wilkins at LWW.com/medstudent.

We owe much gratitude to the contributing authors Ekokobe Fonkem, Chioma A. Ezeadichie, Jameelah Harris, and Roxanna Rodriguez for their time and unfailing effort. We would also like to thank Donna Balado, Cheryl Stringfellow, and Tenille Sands for their encouragement to undertake this text to completion. Without their unconditional support and enduring work, this endeavor could have never happened.

Dai Kohara
Andrew D. Mosier

Contributors

Chioma A. Ezeadichie
New York College of Osteopathic
  Medicine
New York, New York
Chapters 2, 5

Ekokobe Fonkem
St Joseph's Hospital
Warren, Ohio
Chapters 3, 6

Jameelah Harris
Doctor's Hospital
Columbus, Ohio
Chapters 7, 12

Roxanna Rodriguez
Doctor's Hospital
Columbus, Ohio
Chapters 10, 11

Contents

Chapter 1

The Basics of Osteopathy

What are A.T. Still's four osteopathic principles?

1. The body is a unit.
2. The body possesses self-regulatory mechanisms.
3. Structure and function are reciprocally interrelated.
4. Rational therapy is based on an understanding of the first three principles.

1.10

What is the American Osteopathic Association's (AOA) definition of somatic dysfunction?

An impairment or altered function among related components of the body, including skeletal, arthroidal, and myofascial structures, in addition to related vascular, lymphatic, and neural elements.

1.567

What is allostasis?

A bodily state that deviates from homeostasis, increasing activity of the neuroendocrine-immune network in response to any threat (i.e., disease, distress); the state of allostasis is supported by arousal of the sympathetic nervous system with increased levels of noradrenaline and cortisol.

1.150

What does TART stand for when diagnosing osteopathic somatic dysfunction?

1. **T**issue texture changes
2. **A**symmetry
3. **R**estriction
4. **T**enderness

1.557, 1.562

What are tissue texture changes?

Edema, tenderness, hypertrophy, atrophy, rigidity, bogginess, stringiness

1.562

What is restriction?

A joint with limited motion

1.562

What is the only subjective component of the TART criteria for somatic dysfunction?

Tenderness is the only subjective component of the TART criteria for somatic dysfunction.

1.562, 1.634

What is tenderness?

A discomforting or painful area of tissue and the surrounding area of somatic dysfunction

1.562

What three types of barriers can an osteopathic physician encounter when searching for restriction using the TART criteria?

Anatomic (physiologic), restrictive (pathologic), and elastic (which is the range between the physiologic and anatomic barrier of motion in which passive ligamentous stretching occurs before tissue disruption)

1.634

What is an anatomic barrier?

The point a physician or external force can passively move a given joint to, but not beyond, without potential harm; this can be thought of as the limit of passive motion.

1.634

What is a physiologic barrier?

The limit of active motion

1.634

What is a restrictive (pathologic) barrier?

A functional limit within the anatomic motion, which abnormally decreases the normal physiologic range

1.634, 12.8

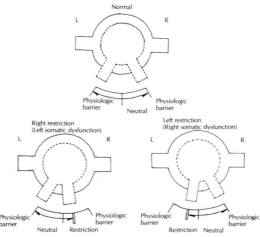

Figure 1–1.

What is tissue bogginess?	A tissue texture abnormality characterized by a palpable sense of sponginess in the surrounding tissues, resulting from congestion due to increased fluid content	12.8
What is ropiness?	A tissue texture abnormality characterized by a cordlike or stringlike feeling	12.8
What is stringiness?	A tissue texture abnormality characterized by palpable string-like myofascial structures	12.8

Using the TART criteria:

What type of tissue texture changes take place in acute somatic dysfunction?	Vasodilation, inflammation, warm and moist skin, increased muscle tone, edema, and bogginess	1.562
What type of tissue texture changes take place in chronic somatic dysfunction?	Cool and pale skin, decreased muscle tone, doughy tissue texture, stringiness, and fibrotic changes	1.562
What type of asymmetric change takes place in acute somatic dysfunction?	A visibly noticeable asymmetry often with a history of recent injury	1.562
What type of asymmetric change takes place in chronic somatic dysfunction?	A long-standing asymmetry that is less visibly noticeable because other body structures have compensated for the acute asymmetry	1.562, 1.634
What type of restriction takes place in acute somatic dysfunction?	An acutely sluggish restriction, often with a relatively normal range of motion	1.562
What type of restriction takes place in chronic somatic dysfunction?	Limited range of motion	1.562
What types of tenderness are felt in acute somatic dysfunction?	Severe, cutting, and sharp	1.562

What types of tenderness are felt in chronic somatic dysfunction?

Dull, achy, crawling, itching, burning, and gnawing

1.562

In acute somatic dysfunction, what happens to the temperature of the area surrounding the dysfunctional tissue?

The temperature increases.

12.8

In acute somatic dysfunction, what happens to the moisture of the surrounding dysfunctional tissue?

The moisture surrounding the dysfunctional tissue increases.

12.8

In acute somatic dysfunction, describe the tension of the dysfunctional tissue.

The tension is increased, and the tissue feels rigid and boardlike to the examiner.

12.8

In acute somatic dysfunction, is edema present?

Yes; edema of the dysfunctional tissue is present.

12.8

In acute somatic dysfunction, what happens when an erythema test (red reflex) is performed?

The redness lasts.

12.8

In chronic somatic dysfunction, what happens to the temperature of the area surrounding the dysfunctional tissue?

A slight increase in temperature is possible; however, a palpable sense of coolness is more likely felt by the examiner.

12.8

In chronic somatic dysfunction, what happens to the moisture of the surrounding dysfunctional tissue?

It is absent and the surrounding dysfunctional tissue is dry.

12.8

In chronic somatic dysfunction, describe the tension of the dysfunctional tissue.

The tension is slightly increased, and the tissue feels ropy and stringy to the examiner.

12.8

In chronic somatic dysfunction, is edema present?	**No;** although edema of the dysfunctional tissue is present in acute somatic dysfunction, it is usually *not* present in chronic somatic dysfunction.	12.8
In chronic somatic dysfunction, what happens when an erythema test (red reflex) is performed?	The redness fades quickly or blanching occurs.	12.8
What is a vertebral unit?	Two adjacent vertebra and their associated arthroidal, ligamentous, muscular, vascular, neural, and lymphatic elements	1.569
What is a vertebral segment?	A single vertebra	1.569
True or False: All vertebral motions (flexion, extension, sidebending (one word in style sheet) rotation, etc.) are described by how the anterior and superior surfaces of a vertebra move in relation to the vertebra below.	**True;** this is a simple but easily and often confused basic concept.	1.569
How is somatic dysfunction recorded by the physician: to the direction of ease or to the direction of dysfunction?	Somatic dysfunction is always recorded to the direction of ease, the direction that the vertebra or dysfunctional joint can move most freely.	1.569
What is a direct treatment?	A technique where the dysfunctional joint is positioned into restriction "against its barrier"	12.13
What is the goal of a direct treatment?	To use force in such a way that motion will be created through and beyond the restrictive barrier	12.13

What is an indirect treatment?	A technique where the dysfunctional joint is positioned in the direction where it most freely moves, away from the barrier or restriction of motion	12.13
What is the goal of an indirect treatment?	To allow the body's inherent neurologic or intrinsic forces to free up the restriction of motion so that the joint will regain its ability to move freely through the restrictive barrier	12.13
Is a myofascial release treatment technique direct or indirect?	Both; at times it is direct, at other times it can be used indirectly.	12.14–15
Is a ligamentous articular strain treatment technique direct or indirect?	Both; at times it is direct, at other times it can be used indirectly.	12.14–15
Is a counterstrain treatment technique direct or indirect?	Indirect	12.14–15
Is a facilitated positional release treatment technique direct or indirect?	Indirect	12.14–15
Is a muscle energy treatment technique direct or indirect?	Direct (rarely it can be used in an indirect manner)	12.14–15
Is an HVLA (high velocity, low amplitude a.k.a. mobilization with impulse) treatment technique direct or indirect?	Direct	**12.14, 12.15**
Is a cranial treatment technique direct or indirect?	Both; at times it is direct, at other times it can be used indirectly.	12.14–15
When treating lymphatics, is the treatment direct or indirect?	Direct	12.14–15

When treating a Chapman reflex, is the treatment direct or indirect?	Direct	12.14–15
Is a myofascial release treatment technique active or passive?	Both; at times it is active, at other times it can be used in a passive manner.	12.14–15
Is a ligamentous articular strain treatment technique active or passive?	Both; at times it is active, at other times it can be used in a passive manner	12.14–15
Is a counterstrain treatment technique active or passive?	Passive	12.14–15
Is a facilitated positional release treatment technique active or passive?	Passive	12.14–15
Is a muscle energy treatment technique active or passive?	Active	12.14–15
Is an HVLA treatment technique active or passive?	Passive	12.14–15
Is a cranial treatment technique active or passive?	Passive	12.14–15
When treating lymphatics, is the treatment active or passive?	Passive	12.14–15
When treating a Chapman reflex, is the treatment active or passive?	Passive	12.14–15
What osteopathic treatments are direct?	1. Chapman reflexes 2. Lymphatic 3. HVLA 4. Muscle energy	12.14–15
What is the only osteopathic treatment that is always an active treatment?	Muscle energy	12.14–15

To what two regions of the spine do Fryette Laws apply?	Fryette laws applies to the thoracic and lumbar spines.	1.569
What is another name for type I motion in Fryette's first law?	Neutral mechanics	1.569
In type I motion, does sidebending or rotation occur first?	Sidebending occurs first.	1.571
Are type I motion dysfunctions associated more with group dysfunctions or dysfunction of a single vertebra?	Group dysfunctions	1.569–571
In type I motion, does the spine prefer flexion and extension or neutrality?	The spine prefers neutrality.	1.571
In type I motion do sidebending and rotation take place in the same direction or opposite directions?	They take place in opposite directions.	1.571
How would a type I motion dysfunction be written if T10 was restricted in left sidebending?	T10 NS_RR_L	1.569–571
In type II motion, does sidebending or rotation occur first?	Rotation occurs first.	1.571
Are type II motion dysfunctions associated more with group dysfunctions or dysfunction of a single vertebra?	A single vertebra	1.571
In type II motion, does the spine prefer flexion/extension or neutrality?	The spine prefers **flexion/ extension.**	1.571

In type II motion, do sidebending and rotation take place in the same direction or opposite directions?

They take place in the same direction.

1.571

How would a type II motion dysfunction be written if T10 were restricted in left sidebending?

T10 ER_RS_R or T10 FR_RS_R, depending on whether the dysfunction was flexed or extended

1.571

Summarize Fryette's first law of spinal mechanics.

1. Neutral mechanics
2. Sidebending before rotation in opposite directions
3. Restricted in the coronal plane
4. Group dysfunctions

1.571

Summarize Fryette's second law of spinal mechanics.

1. Nonneutral mechanics
2. Rotation before sidebending in the same direction
3. No longer restricted in the sagittal plane
4. Single-vertebra dysfunction

1.571

How does the spine appear clinically to an examining physician when a type I dysfunction is present?

With a lateral curvature to the spine

12.56

Is the onset of pain in a type I dysfunction abrupt or gradual?

The onset of pain is usually gradual.

12.56

Where is the site of pain usually elicited when palpating for a type I dysfunction?

Pain can be elicited on either the convex side (because of the stretched paraspinal musculature) or the concave side (because of the contracted paraspinal musculature).

12.56

How does the spine appear clinically to an examining physician when a type II dysfunction is present?

With either a flattening *or* exaggeration of the anteroposterior (AP) spinal curve

12.56

Is the onset of pain in a type II dysfunction abrupt or gradual?	The onset of pain is usually abrupt, occurring concurrently with the injury.	12.56
Where is the site of pain usually elicited when palpating for a type II dysfunction?	Usually over the most posterior facet	12.56
What is passive motion?	Motion induced by the physician with the patient remaining passive or relaxed	1.571
What is active motion?	Patient-initiated, voluntary motion	1.571
What type of information does passive motion testing of a vertebral unit provide?	Quantity, direction, and end-feel of motion in each of the three cardinal planes of motion	1.571
What type of information does active motion testing of a vertebral unit provide?	An assessment of the vertebral unit's combined ease and restriction of motion; this is accomplished by palpating over the transverse process as the patient flexes or extends outside of the "easy and free" neutral range.	1.571
What does Fryette's third law of spinal motion describe?	Movement in one of the three cardinal directions of motion (flexion/extension, sidebending (see style sheet), and rotation) limits the motion of the other two cardinal directions of motion; for example, sidebending a segment to the right will limit the amount of flexion/extension and rotation a segment would normally be capable of moving.	12.57
Which directions are the facets oriented in the cervical spine?	Backward, upward, and medial	12.75–76

Which directions are the facets oriented in the thoracic spine?	Backward, upward, and lateral	✎	12.76
Which directions are the facets oriented in the lumbar spine?	Backward and medial	✎	12.76
In what axis of motion does flexion and extension of the spine take place?	The transverse axis		9.5–12
In what axis of motion does sidebending of the spine take place?	The anterior-posterior axis		9.5–12
In what axis of motion does rotation of the spine take place?	The vertical axis		9.5–12
In what plane of motion does flexion and extension of the spine take place?	The sagittal plane		9.5–12
In what plane of motion does sidebending of the spine take place?	The coronal plane		9.5–12
In what plane of motion does rotation of the spine take place?	The transverse plane		9.5–12
A sicker patient should be treated with a greater or lesser dosage (amount and duration) of osteopathic manipulative therapy (OMT)?	The sicker the patient, the less the dose; caring and compassionate new D.O.'s often err on the side of overdosing/overtreating. Do not forget to allow sufficient time for the patient to respond to the treatment.		1.577
Should pediatric patients be treated more or less frequently?	Pediatric patients can be treated more frequently; however, as with all fields of medicine, clinical judgment should be carefully applied.		1.577

Should geriatric patients be treated more or less frequently?	Geriatric patients need a longer interval to respond to treatment and should therefore be treated less frequently; however, as with all fields of medicine, clinical judgment should be carefully applied.	1.577
How should acute cases of somatic dysfunction be treated with regard to frequency of treatment?	Acute cases should have a shorter interval between treatments; as the patient responds, the interval can be increased.	1.577
What part of the spine should be treated first in low back complaints where the psoas is presumed to be involved?	The thoracic spine	1.577
What two body regions should be treated before treating the cervical spine?	Treat the upper thoracic spine and ribs before treating the cervical spine.	1.577
Should a physician treat the ribs or the thoracic spine first?	Treatment of the thoracic spine is recommended before treatment of specific rib dysfunctions.	1.577
True of False: For acute somatic dysfunctions, focus your treatment immediately on the dysfunctional area to prevent further damage to the tissues.	False; for very acute somatic dysfunction, treat the secondary and peripheral areas first to allow access to the acute area.	1.577
What type of osteopathic treatment may relax the patient and allow OMT to be more effective in other areas of the body?	Cranial techniques (discussed in Chapter 12 with further detail)	1.577
How should a physician approach treatment of somatic dysfunction in the arms and legs?	The physician should treat the axial skeletal components first and then reassess the extremities for the best possible ensuing treatment.	1.577

Chapter 2

The Human Spine, Rib Cage, and Sacrum

Cervical Spine

Which cervical vertebrae are considered atypical?	C1, because it has no spinous process or vertebral body, and C2, because it has a dens	9.1047
What cervical vertebrae are considered typical?	C3-C6, because they all have bifid spinous processes, facets, articular pillars, a vertebral body, and foramen transversariums	9.1047
What is the clinical significance of the articular pillars?	They are used to evaluate cervical motion and are located between the superior and inferior facets.	1.688
What is the function of the scalene muscles?	They sidebend the neck ipsilaterally with unilateral contraction and flex the neck with bilateral contraction.	9.1026–1027
What are the attachments for the scalene muscles?	The anterior and middle scalenes attach to rib 1 and help to elevate this rib during forced inhalation. The posterior scalene attaches to rib 2 and helps to elevate this rib during forced inhalation.	9.1057–1058
What muscle divides the neck into anterior and posterior triangles?	The sternocleidomastoid muscle	9.1053–1055
Torticollis results from shortening or restriction of which muscle(s)?	The sternocleidomastoid muscle	9.1055–1056

Which conditions can weaken the alar and transverse ligaments causing atlantoaxial (AA) subluxation?	Rheumatoid arthritis and Down syndrome	3.209
What are the most common causes of cervical nerve root compression?	Degeneration of the joints of Luschka and hypertrophic arthritis of facet joints	3.212, 3.219
What are the signs and symptoms of intervertebral foraminal stenosis?	1. Neck pain radiating to the upper extremity 2. Increased pain with neck extension 3. A positive Spurling test 4. Paraspinal muscle spasm 5. Cervical tenderpoints	3.219–3.220
How many cervical nerve roots are there?	Eight nerve roots C1-C7 exit above their corresponding vertebrae. C8 exits between C7 and T1.	13.330
Do Fryette's first and second laws apply to cervical vertebrae?	**No;** they apply only to the thoracic and lumbar vertebrae.	1.571, 1.1242–1243
Flexion and extension is the main motion for which cervical segment?	The occipitoatlantal (OA) joint *Note:* The OA joint is known as the "yes joint" because it nods the head forward and back, as if shaking your head *yes*.	3.188
Rotation is the main motion for which cervical segments?	The AA joint along with C2-C4 *Note:* AA is known as the "no joint" because it rotates the head from side to side, as if shaking your head *no*.	3.189
Sidebending is the main motion of which cervical segments?	The C5-C7 segments	3.189

Do the OA and AA joints sidebend and rotate in the same direction or opposite directions?

The OA and AA joints sidebend and rotate in **opposite directions.**

3.188–3.189

Do the C2-C7 cervical segments sidebend and rotate in the same direction or opposite directions?

The C2-C7 cervical segments sidebend and rotate to the **same side.**

3.188–189

Translation of C3 to the right corresponds with which direction of sidebending?

Translation and sidebending are opposite of each other; therefore, right translation of C3 corresponds with sidebending C3 to the left.

3.579–580

How is rotation at the AA joint tested?

By flexing the neck to 45°, because after the cervical spine has been flexed to 45°, rotation at all other cervical joints from C2-C7 is locked out.

3.582–583

What initial treatments to the cervical spine are best indicated for acute injury?

1. Indirect facial release
2. Counterstrain
3. Cranial techniques

1.688

Thoracic Spine

Which thoracic segments' spinous processes are located at about the same level as their corresponding transverse processes?

Levels T1-T3, T12

1.715

Which thoracic segments' spinous processes are located about one-half segment below their corresponding transverse processes?

Levels T4-T6, T11

1.715

Which thoracic segments' spinous processes are located about one entire segment below their corresponding transverse processes?

Levels T7-T9, T10

1.715

The sternal notch corresponds to which thoracic vertebrae?	The level of the T2 vertebra	9.83
What dermatome level is associated with the nipples?	The T4 dermatome	9.51–53
The spine of scapula corresponds to which thoracic vertebrae?	The level of the T3 vertebra	9.83
The inferior angle of the scapula corresponds to which thoracic vertebrae?	The level of the T7 vertebra	9.83
What dermatome level is associated with the umbilicus?	The T10 dermatome	9.51–9.53
The sternal angle of Louis corresponds to which thoracic vertebrae?	The level of the T4 vertebra	9.83, 13.141
What is the main motion of the thoracic spine—flexion/extension, sidebending, or rotation?	The main motion of the thoracic spine is rotation.	1.713
Do Fryette's laws apply to the thoracic spine?	**Yes;** Fryette's first, second, and third laws apply to the thoracic and lumbar spines.	1.1242–1243

Rib Cage

What are the primary muscles of respiration?	The diaphragm and intercostal muscles	9.93–98
What are the secondary muscles of respiration?	1. Scalenes 2. Pectoralis minor 3. Serratus anterior and posterior 4. Quadratus lumborum 5. Latissimus dorsi	9.93–9.98

What are the attachments of the diaphragm?	1. Xiphoid process 2. Ribs 6 through 12 3. L1-L3 vertebral bodies 4. Intervertebral discs	13.234–235
What ribs are considered the typical ribs?	Ribs 3 through 9, because they have a head, neck, tubercle, angle, and shaft	13.142
What ribs are considered the atypical ribs?	1. Rib 1, because it has no angle and articulates only with T1 2. Rib 2, because of the large tuberosity on its shaft for the serratus anterior muscle 3. Ribs 11 and 12, because they have no tubercles and articulate only with their corresponding vertebrae 4. Rib 10 is sometimes considered atypical because it articulates only with T10. For boards, know that any rib with a 1 or 2 in its number is considered atypical.	13.142
What ribs are referred to as the true ribs?	Ribs 1 through 7, because they attach to the sternum via the costal cartilages	13.142
What ribs are referred to as the false ribs?	Ribs 8 through 12 (because they do not attach directly to sternum, but are connected by costal cartilages to the cartilage of the rib above)	13.142

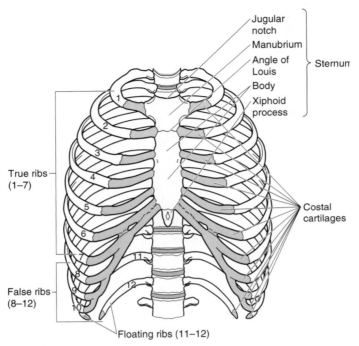

Figure 2–1.

What ribs are referred to as the floating ribs?	Ribs 11 and 12, because they do not attach to the sternum	13.142
Pump handle motion is the primary motion of which ribs?	Ribs 2 through 5	9.89–90, 1.720–722
Which ribs move primarily with a bucket handle motion?	Ribs 6 through 10	9.89–90, 1.720–722
Which ribs move primarily with a caliper-like motion?	Ribs 11 and 12	1.720–722

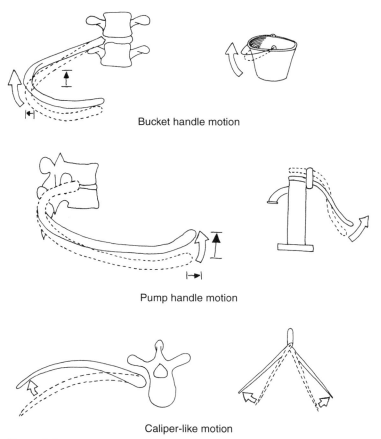

Bucket handle motion

Pump handle motion

Caliper-like motion

Figure 2–2.

To varying degrees, do all ribs exhibit each of the three types of characteristic rib motion (pump handle, bucket handle, and caliper-like)?	**Yes; although** ribs can be grouped by the primary type of motion they demonstrate, including pump handle, bucket handle, and caliper-like, all ribs to varying degrees exhibit each of the three types of characteristic rib motion.	1.720– 722
What are the most common types of rib dysfunction?	Inhalation and exhalation rib dysfunctions	1.1245

What are the characteristics of an inhalation dysfunction rib?	The dysfunctional rib will move cephalad during inhalation but will not move caudad during exhalation; this indicates that the rib is **stuck upward.**	1.724, 1.1245
What are the diagnostic findings of an inhalation dysfunction pump handle rib?	1. The rib is elevated anteriorly. 2. The anterior rib moves cephalad and is stuck on inspiration. 3. Anterior narrowing of intercostal space above the dysfunctional rib. 4. A prominent posterior rib angle.	4.123, 4.129
What are the diagnostic findings of an inhalation dysfunction bucket handle rib?	1. The rib is elevated laterally. 2. The shaft moves cephalad and is stuck on inspiration. 3. Lateral narrowing of intercostal space above the dysfunctional rib occurs. 4. There is a prominent rib shaft.	4.123, 4.129
What are the characteristics of an exhalation dysfunction rib?	The dysfunctional rib will move caudad during exhalation but will not move cephalad during inhalation; this indicates that the rib is **stuck downward.**	1.724, 1.1245
What are the diagnostic findings of an exhalation dysfunction pump handle rib?	1. The rib is depressed anteriorly. 2. The anterior rib moves caudad and is stuck on expiration. 3. Anterior narrowing of intercostal space below the dysfunctional rib occurs. 4. There is a prominent posterior rib angle.	4.126, 4.131
What are the diagnostic findings of an exhalation dysfunction bucket handle rib?	1. The rib is depressed laterally. 2. The rib shaft moves caudad and is stuck on expiration. 3. Lateral narrowing of intercostal space below the dysfunctional rib occurs.	4.126, 4.131

What is a key rib?	A rib that is "stuck" (little mobility or immobile); this rib is usually considered the rib that causes the group dysfunction.	1.723
In an inhalation group dysfunction, which rib is the key rib?	The **lowest rib** of the dysfunction	1.723–724
In an exhalation group dysfunction, which rib is the key rib?	The **uppermost rib** of the dysfunction	1.723–724
In a group dysfunction, treatment is directed at which rib?	The key rib	1.723
Which muscles are targeted for a muscle energy technique when treating a first rib dysfunction?	The anterior and middle scalenes	3.565
When treating a dysfunction of rib 2 with muscle energy, what muscle is targeted?	The posterior scalene muscle	3.565
When treating a dysfunction of ribs 3 through 5 with muscle energy, what muscle is targeted?	Pectoralis minor	3.565
When treating a dysfunction of ribs 6 through 9 with muscle energy, what muscle is targeted?	Serratus anterior	3.565
When treating a dysfunction of ribs 10 and 11 with muscle energy, what muscle is targeted?	Latissimus dorsi	3.565
When treating a dysfunction of rib 12 with muscle energy, what muscle is targeted?	Quadratus lumborum	3.565

Lumbar Spine

True or False: At L4 and L5, the posterior longitudinal ligament is half the width that it is at L1.	**True;** this ligament narrows as it descends to the lumbar area, producing a weakness in the posteriolateral aspect of the intervertebral disc, making the lumbar spine more susceptible to disc herniation, most commonly in the posteriolateral direction.	3.250
Where does the L3 nerve root exit the spinal column?	It exits between L3 and L4.	9.518–520
A herniation at L3-L4 will compress what nerve root?	The L4 nerve root	9.518–521
What is the most common anomaly in the lumbar spine?	Facet trophism	3.449
In what lumbar spinal condition would the transverse processes of L5 be long and abnormally articulate with the sacrum?	The lumbar spinal condition known as *sacralization*	9.494
In what lumbar spinal condition does S1 fail to fuse with the other sacral segments?	The lumbar spinal condition known as *lumbarization*	9.494
What bony structure is defective in spina bifida occulta?	The lamina of L5 (and/or S1), because it fails to develop and fuse	13.316, 9.494–496
What bony structure is defective in spina bifida cystica?	One or more of the vertebral arches, because they fail to develop	13.316, 9.494–496
Which type of spina bifida is associated with neurological deficits?	A meningomyelocele (herniation of the meninges and spinal cord)	13.316, 9.494–496

What is the main motion of the lumbar spine?

The main motion of the lumbar spine is **flexion/extension.**

1.737–738

How does motion at L5 influence sacral motion?

1. Sidebending of L5 engages the **ipsilateral** sacral oblique axis.
2. Rotation of L5 causes rotation of sacrum to **opposite side.**

1.780

What are some prominent signs and symptoms of back strain/sprain?

1. Achy pain in the low back, buttock, or posterior-lateral thigh
2. Increased pain with activity, prolonged standing, or sitting
3. Increased muscle tension

9.478

What are some prominent signs and symptoms of a herniated disc?

1. Numbness; tingling; and sharp, burning, and/or shooting pain in the lower back, radiating down the leg *beyond* the knee; worsens with flexion of the lumbar spine
2. Weakness
3. Decreased deep tendon reflexes (DTRs)
4. Sensory loss associated with the nerve root

6.276

What test can be performed to check for disc herniation?

A straight-leg raising test; the test is positive if pain radiates beyond the knee.

1.488

How is a herniated disc typically managed?

Bed rest and indirect osteopathic manipulative therapy (OMT) techniques, followed by gentle direct techniques; **very few herniations require surgery.**

6.276

What are the more common causes of iliopsoas syndrome?

1. Prolonged positions that shorten the psoas muscle
2. Appendicitis
3. Ureteral calculi
4. Salpingitis
5. Prostatitis
6. Sigmoid colon dysfunction
7. Ureter dysfunction

1.748, 3.484

What are some prominent signs and symptoms of iliopsoas syndrome?

1. Achy or spasmic low back pain that sometimes radiates to the groin
2. Increased pain when standing or walking
3. L1 or L2 FRS (flexed, rotated, and sidebent) to same side
4. Positive pelvic shift test to the contralateral side
5. Contralateral piriformis spasm
6. Sacral dysfunction on an oblique axis

1.747–748

What test can be performed to check for iliopsoas syndrome?

A Thomas test that is positive if the patient's tight hip flexors will not allow the affected leg to completely straighten out when the opposite leg is flexed to the chest with the patient in a supine position

1.743

How do you treat iliopsoas syndrome?

1. Ice to decrease edema and pain
2. Counterstrain to the anterior iliopsoas tenderpoint
3. Muscle energy or high velocity, low amplitude (HVLA) to L1 or L2

1.748, 3.488–489

Degenerative changes in the lumbar spine, such as hypertrophy of facet joints, loss of intervertebral disc height, and calcium deposits within ligaments, can lead to what spinal condition?

Spinal stenosis, a condition that can lead to nerve root compression

9.489–490

What are some prominent signs and symptoms of spinal stenosis?

Achy, shooting pain, or paresthesias in the low back that radiates to the lower leg, along with pain that is worsened by lower extremity extension (standing, walking, or lying supine)

3.575, 6.277

What radiographic findings are commonly present in spinal stenosis?	Osteophytes and a decreased intervertebral disc space	3.575
How is spinal stenosis usually managed?	1. OMT to decrease any restrictions and improve range of motion 2. Physical therapy 3. Nonsteroidal anti-inflammatory drugs (NSAIDs) or low-dose steroids 4. If needed, epidural steroid injections or a surgical decompressive laminectomy	6.277
What is spondylolisthesis?	Anterior displacement of one vertebra in relation to the vertebrae below owing to fracture of par interarticularis; it often occurs at L4 or L5.	1.1250
What are some prominent signs and symptoms of spondylolisthesis?	1. Achy pain in low back, buttock, or posterior thigh 2. Increased pain with extension 3. Tight hamstrings bilaterally 4. Positive vertebral step-off sign *Note:* Half of all patients with spondylolisthesis are asymptomatic.	3.366–367, 1.625, 1.627
What radiographic findings are commonly present in spondylolisthesis?	Anterior displacement of one vertebra on another seen with lateral x-rays of the lumbar spine	3.366–367
What is spondylolysis?	Fracture of the pars interarticularis **without** anterior displacement of a vertebral body	13.315, 13.320, 1.490
What radiographic findings are commonly present in spondylolysis?	Oblique x-rays of the lumbar spine will show what resembles a "collar on the neck of a Scottie dog" sign.	6.278

What is spondylosis?	**Degenerative changes** within the intervertebral disc and ankylosis of adjacent vertebral bodies	1.1251, 13.315, 13.320
What radiographic findings are commonly present in spondylosis?	Lipping of the vertebral bodies	6.278
What causes cauda equina syndrome?	A large central disc herniation that exerts pressure on the nerve roots of the cauda equina	1.744, 6.276
What are some prominent signs and symptoms of cauda equina syndrome?	1. Saddle anesthesia 2. Decreased DTRs 3. Loss of bowel and bladder control	1.744, 6.276
Is surgery required for treatment of cauda equina syndrome?	**Yes;** emergency surgery is necessary and if delayed may lead to irreversible paralysis.	1.744

Scoliosis and Short Leg Syndrome

How is scoliosis named?	A curve that is sidebent left causes scoliosis to the right, known as **dextroscoliosis,** and a curve that is sidebent right causes scoliosis to the left, known as **levoscoliosis.**	6.226
What type of spinal curve is flexible and can be corrected with sidebending or rotation?	A functional curve: A **F**unctional spinal curve can be **F**ixed.	1.619, 6.227
What type of spinal curve will not correct with sidebending or rotation?	A structural curve: You are **ST**uck with a **ST**ructural spinal curve.	1.619, 6.226–227
How do you measure scoliotic curves?	By evaluating the Cobb angle on an x-ray	1.620, 6.227

Curvature

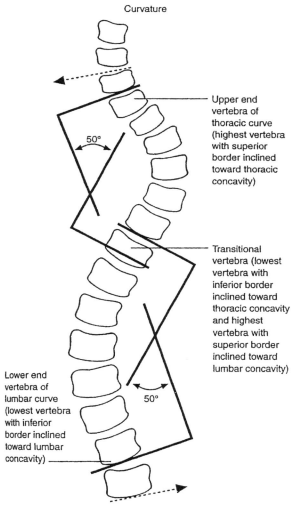

Upper end vertebra of thoracic curve (highest vertebra with superior border inclined toward thoracic concavity)

Transitional vertebra (lowest vertebra with inferior border inclined toward thoracic concavity and highest vertebra with superior border inclined toward lumbar concavity)

Lower end vertebra of lumbar curve (lowest vertebra with inferior border inclined toward lumbar concavity)

Figure 2–3.

What is the most common cause of scoliosis?	Idiopathic; other causes include congenital, neuromuscular, and acquired	3.351, 1.619

How is scoliosis usually managed?	1. For *mild* scoliosis: Physical therapy, Konstancin exercises, and **osteopathic manipulative therapy (OMT).** 2. For *moderate* scoliosis: The treatment for mild scoliosis **in addition** to spinal orthotic bracing. 3. For *severe* scoliosis: Surgery is indicated.	1.622, 3.339, 3.354
What are some prominent signs and symptoms of short leg syndrome?	1. The sacral base is lower on the side of the short leg. 2. Anterior innominate rotation ipsilaterally. 3. Posterior innominate rotation contralaterally. 4. An increased Ferguson's angle. 5. The lumbar spine will sidebend away and rotate toward the short leg side.	3.344
What is the most common cause of an anatomic leg length discrepancy?	The total hip replacement is the most common cause of an anatomic leg length discrepancy.	3.343
How is short leg syndrome usually managed?	OMT to spine and lower extremity; if the femoral head height difference is >5 mm, consider a heel lift.	3.346

Sacrum and Innominates

What three bones make up the innominate?	1. Illium 2. Ischium 3. Pubis	1.762
What parts of the sacrum are relevant for diagnosing sacral dysfunction?	The sacral base, sacral sulci, inferior lateral angles (ILA) of the sacrum, and the PSIS	1.780–781, 6.313

Which ligaments help to stabilize the sacroiliac (SI) joint?	The sacroiliac ligaments (anterior, posterior, and interosseous)	3.406
Testing the tension of which ligament aids in diagnosing somatic dysfunction of the sacrum?	The sacrotuberous ligament, which runs from the ILA to the ischial tuberosity	3.407
Which ligament divides the greater and lesser sciatic foramen?	The sacrospinous ligament, which runs from the sacrum to the ischial spine	3.407
In lumbosacral decompensation which ligament is often the first to become painful?	The iliolumbar ligament	3.407
Where does the iliolumbar ligament attach?	It originates from the L4 and L5 transverse processes and attaches to the medial side of the iliac crest.	3.407
What muscles make up the pelvic diaphragm?	The levator ani and the coccygeus muscles	3.408
In some people, the sciatic nerve runs through what muscle?	The piriformis muscle	3.408
Hypertonicity of what muscle can cause buttock pain that radiates down the thigh without reaching the knee?	The piriformis muscle	3.408
What motions occur around the superior transverse axis of the sacrum located at S2?	Respiratory motion and craniosacral (inherent) motion	1.768, 3.401

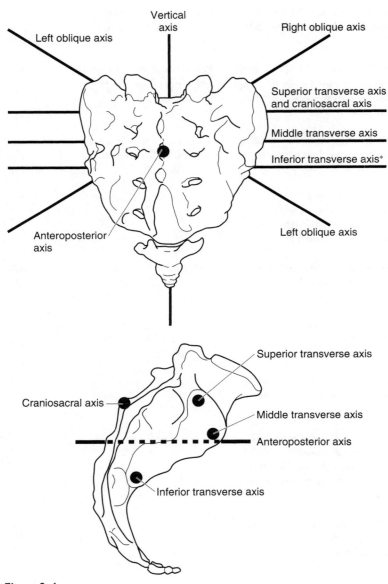

Figure 2–4.

What motion occurs around the middle transverse axis of the sacrum?	Postural-type motion	1.768
What motion occurs around the inferior axis of the sacrum?	Innominate rotation (during walking)	1.768
While walking (dynamic motion), what causes a left sacral oblique axis to be engaged?	Weight bearing on the left leg while stepping forward with the right leg	1.768
A positive standing flexion test is used for the diagnosis of what type of dysfunction?	An innominate dysfunction	6.305
What type of dysfunction occurs when a tight quadriceps muscle causes an innominate to rotate more anteriorly compared to the other?	Anterior innominate dysfunction	1.777, 4.219
If the standing flexion test is positive on the right, the right ASIS is more inferior, and the right PSIS is more superior, what is the diagnosis?	Right anterior innominate dysfunction	1.777, 4.219
What type of dysfunction occurs when a tight hamstring muscle causes an innominate to rotate more posteriorly compared to the other?	Posterior innominate dysfunction	1.777, 4.214
If the standing flexion test is positive on the left, the right ASIS is more superior, and the right PSIS is more inferior, what is the diagnosis?	Left posterior innominate dysfunction	1.777, 4.214

If the standing flexion test is positive on the right, the right ASIS and PSIS are more superior, the right pubic rami is more superior, and the right leg appears shorter, what is the diagnosis?	Right innominate upslip, also known as a right superior innominate shear (Table 2-1)	1.778, 4.223, 6.310–311
If the standing flexion test is positive on the right, the right ASIS and PSIS are more inferior, the right pubic rami is more inferior, and the right leg appears longer, what is the diagnosis?	Right innominate downslip, also known as a right inferior innominate shear	1.778, 6.310–311
A tight rectus abdominus muscle causing an ipsilateral pubic bone to be displaced superiorly is known as what?	A superior pubic shear	1.778, 4.185
Tight adductors that pull the ipsilateral pubic bone inferiorly can lead to what type of dysfunction?	An inferior pubic shear	1.778, 4.187
What types of dysfunctions occur about the sacral oblique axes?	Sacral torsions	1.778–779
True or False: The seated flexion test is positive on the opposite side of the engaged sacral oblique axis.	**True;** therefore if the seated flexion test is positive on the right, the left sacral oblique axis is engaged.	1.773, 1.779
If L5 is ER_RS_R, on what side is the seated flexion test positive?	On the left side	1.780–781
If L5 is NS_RR_L, what is the sacral diagnosis?	The sacrum would be rotated right on a right oblique axis (R on R).	1.780–781

Table 2-1.

Static Findings					Tests			Results	
ILA Posterior	Deep Sulcus	Shallow Sulcus	L5 Rotation	Seated Flexion	Lumbar Spring	Sphinx Test	Diagnosis	Axis
Right	Right	Left		Right	Negative	Negative	Right unilateral shear	
Left	Left	Right		Left	Negative	Negative	Left unilateral shear	
Right	Left	Right	Right	Left	Negative	Negative	Right on right (R on R) rotation	Right oblique
Right	Left	Right	Left	Left	Negative	Negative	Right on right (R on R) torsion	Right oblique
Left	Right	Left	Left	Right	Negative	Negative	Left on left (L on L) rotation	Left oblique
Left	Right	Left	Right	Right	Negative	Negative	Left on left (L on L) torsion	Left oblique
Right	Left	Right	Right	Right	Positive	Positive	Right on left (R on L) rotation	Left oblique
Right	Left	Right	Left	Right	Positive	Positive	Right on left (R on L) torsion	Left oblique
Left	Right	Left	Left	Left	Positive	Positive	Left on right (L on R) rotation	Right oblique
Left	Right	Left	Right	Left	Positive	Positive	Left on right (L on R) torsion	Right oblique
Even	Bilateral			Equivocal	Negative	Negative	Bilateral sacral flexion	Transverse
Even		Bilateral		Equivocal	Equivocal		Bilateral sacral extension	Transverse

From DiGiovanna EL, Schiowitz S, Dowling DJ, eds. An Osteopathic Approach to Diagnosis and Treatment. 3rd ed. Philadelphia: Lippincott Williams & Wilkins, 2005:320.

When is a lumbosacral spring test positive?

When the sacral base is posterior

1.781

What two dysfunctions are considered forward sacral torsion?

L on L and R on R

1.778, 4.203

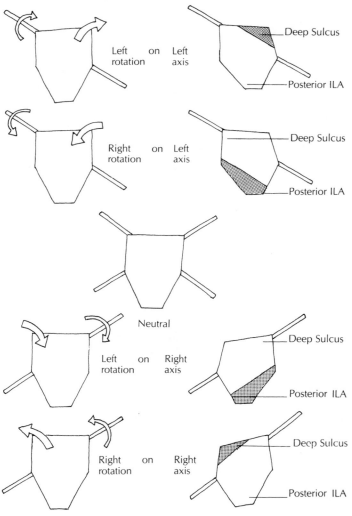

Figure 2–5.

True or False: Forward torsions occur when the lumbar spine is neutral.	**True**	1.780
In a L on L torsion, what landmarks are deep (anterior)?	The right sacral sulcus and the right ILA	1.780, 4.203
What side is the seated flexion test positive on with a L on L sacral torsion?	On the right side	1.780, 4.203
Is the lumbosacral spring test positive or negative with a L on L sacral torsion dysfunction?	The lumbosacral spring test is negative.	4.203
In a R on R torsion, what landmarks are deep (anterior)?	The left sacral sulcus and the left ILA	1.780, 4.203
What side is the seated flexion test positive on with a R on R sacral torsion?	On the left side	1.780, 4.203
Is the lumbosacral spring test positive or negative with a R on R sacral torsion dysfunction?	The lumbosacral spring test is negative.	4.203
What two dysfunctions are considered backward sacral torsion?	L on R and R on L	1.779, 4.208
True or False: Backward torsions occur when the spine is neutral.	**False;** they occur when the spine is demonstrating nonneutral mechanics.	1.780
In a L on R torsion, what landmarks are deep (anterior)?	The right sacral sulcus and the right ILA	1.780–781, 4.208
What side is the seated flexion test positive on with a L on R sacral torsion?	On the left side	1.780, 4.208

Is the lumbosacral spring test (backward bending test) positive or negative with a L on R sacral torsion dysfunction?	The lumbosacral spring test is **positive.**	4.203
What is the diagnosis of L5 if a L on R sacral torsion is present?	NNR_RS_R (NN = nonneutral which could be either flexion or extension)	1.781, 4.203
In a R on L torsion, what landmarks are deep (anterior)?	The left sacral sulcus and the left ILA	1.781, 4.208
What side is the seated flexion test positive on with a R on L sacral torsion?	On the right side	1.780, 4.203
Is the lumbosacral spring test (backward bending test) positive or negative with a R on L sacral torsion dysfunction?	The lumbosacral spring test is **positive.**	4.203
What is the L5 diagnosis on a R on L torsion?	(F or E) NNR_LS_L	1.781, 4.203
With a bilateral sacral flexion dysfunction, how are sacral sulci and ILAs positioned?	Both sacral sulci are deep and both ILAs are shallow.	1.781, 4.191
Is the lumbosacral spring test (backward bending test) positive or negative with a bilateral sacral flexion dysfunction?	The lumbosacral spring test is negative.	1.781, 4.191
Which patients tend to have bilateral sacral flexion dysfunctions?	**Postpartum patients,** because of birth mechanics	1.781

With a bilateral sacral extension dysfunction, how are sacral sulci and ILAs positioned?	Both sacral sulci are shallow and both ILAs are deep.	1.781, 4.195
Is the lumbosacral spring test (backward bending test) positive or negative with a bilateral sacral extension dysfunction?	The lumbosacral spring test is positive.	1.781, 4.195
What happens to the lumbar curve with a bilateral sacral extension dysfunction?	It decreases.	1.781, 4.195
How are unilateral sacral flexion and extension dysfunctions named?	They are named for the side of the positive seated flexion test.	1.781, 4.211
With a right unilateral sacral flexion, what landmarks are deep (anterior)?	The right sacral sulcus and the left ILA	4.211
Is the lumbosacral spring test (backward bending test) positive or negative with a left unilateral sacral flexion dysfunction?	The lumbosacral spring test is negative.	4.211
With a left unilateral sacral extension, what landmarks are deep (anterior)?	The right sulcus and the left ILA	4.213
Is the lumbosacral spring test (backward bending test) positive or negative with a right unilateral sacral extension dysfunction?	The lumbosacral spring test is positive.	4.213
If a patient has both a sacral somatic dysfunction and an L5 somatic dysfunction, which dysfunction should the physician treat first?	L5, because most of the time a sacral dysfunction will resolve once L5 is successfully treated	1.782

Chapter 3

Upper and Lower Extremities

What is the function of the rotator cuff muscles?

Rotator cuff muscles serve to protect the shoulder joint by holding the humerus in the glenoid fossa.

10.824–829

What four muscles make up the rotator cuff?

The four S.I.T.S. muscles:

7.489

1. **S**upraspinatus
2. **I**nfraspinatus
3. **T**eres minor
4. **S**ubscapularis

What is the maximum degree of rotation in the glenohumeral joint?

The glenohumeral joint in active motion can rotate 120°.

6.410–411

What is the maximum degree of motion of scapulothoracic joint?

The scapulothoracic joint can rotate up to 60°.

6.410–411

What is the maximum degree of abduction of the arm?

The arm in active motion can be abducted to 180°, with the glenohumeral joint contributing 120° and the scapulothoracic joint contributing 60°.

6.410–411

List the motions of the clavicle.

The clavicle can glide anterior and posterior, superior and inferior.

6.416

Which shoulder joint is not a true joint?

Of the four shoulder joints—the scapulothoracic, acromioclavicular, sternoclavicular, and glenohumeral—**the scapulothoracic is the only pseudo joint.**

6.411

What is thoracic outlet syndrome?	Thoracic outlet syndrome is compression of the neurovascular bundle (subclavian vein, artery, and brachial plexus) as it exits the thoracic outlet ✎	1.446–447
Where within the thoracic outlet does compression of the neurovascular bundle occur?	Compression of the neurovascular bundle can occur between the clavicle and the first rib; between the scalenes; and between the pectoralis minor and upper ribs.	1.446–447
What is supraspinatus tendonitis?	Impingement of the greater tuberosity against the acromion as the arm is flexed and internally rotated	7.489
How is supraspinatus tendonitis treated?	Ice, rest, and nonsteroidal anti-inflammatory drugs (NSAIDs) are used for the treatment of acute cases, while steroids and osteopathic manipulative therapy (OMT) are used for the treatment of severe cases.	6.467
What artery accompanies the radial nerve in the radial groove?	The profunda brachial artery runs with the radial nerve in the radial groove.	7.510
What artery becomes the axillary artery at the lateral border of the first rib?	The subclavian artery	10.704
What artery runs between the anterior and middle scalenes?	The subclavian artery	10.704
What structure passes anteriorly to the anterior scalene?	The subclavian vein passes anteriorly to the anterior scalenes.	10.706

At what point does the brachial artery split into the radial and ulnar arteries?	The brachial artery divides into the radial and ulna arteries at the bicipital aponeurosis.	7.506
What treatment options can be utilized to relieve lymph congestion of the upper extremity?	Opening the thoracic inlet, redoming the thoracoabdominal diaphragm, and posterior axillary fold techniques can be utilized to relieve lymph congestion in the upper extremity.	7.465
Which plexus supplies all the nerves to the upper extremity?	The brachial plexus supplies all the nerves of the upper extremity.	7.576
What are the spinal cord exit levels of the brachial plexus?	The brachial plexus exits the spinal cords at the C5-T1 levels.	7.576
What is the most common brachial plexus injury?	**Erb-Duchenne** palsy; this results in paralysis of the deltoid, external rotators, biceps, brachioradialis, and supinator muscles.	7.577
What is the nickname for Erb-Duchenne palsy?	"Waiter's tip" palsy	7.577
In Klumpke palsy, what spinal cord levels are injured?	Klumpke palsy results from injury of the **C8-T1 nerve roots,** and paralysis involves the intrinsic muscles of the hand.	7.577
What is the nickname for Klumpke palsy?	"Claw hand" palsy	7.577
What nerve injury results in winging of the scapula?	Injury to the **long thoracic nerve** will cause winging of the scapula.	7.577
What artery supplies the muscle paralyzed in a long thoracic nerve palsy?	The lateral thoracic artery supplies the serratus anterior muscle; this muscle is paralyzed in an injury to the long thoracic nerve.	

What muscle is innervated by the long thoracic nerve?

The anterior serratus muscle is innervated by the long thoracic nerve.

7.577

What nerve is damaged during shoulder dislocation?

The axillary nerve is injured during shoulder dislocation.

5.794

In what direction does humeral dislocation usually occur?

Most humeral dislocations occur in an anterior and inferior direction.

10.793

What upper extremity nerve is most commonly injured?

The radial nerve is the most common nerve injured in the upper extremity; it is usually injured by direct trauma.

10.762

What muscles are affected by injury to the radial nerve?

Injury to the radial nerve results in paralysis of the extensor muscles of the arm.

10.762

What is the name given to a palsy caused by injury to the radial nerve?

A "wrist drop" or "Saturday night" palsy, from falling asleep intoxicated on a park bench and throwing your arm over the seat all night compressing the radial nerve, or "crutch" palsy, from compression of the radial nerve under the arm due to leaning on the crutch for a prolonged period of time

What nerve innervates most of the primary flexors of the hand?

The median nerve innervates all of the primary flexor muscles of the hand except the flexor carpi ulnaris, which is innervated by the ulnar nerve.

10.737

What nerve innervates the supinator muscles?

The primary supinators of the forearm are the biceps, which are innervated by the, musculocutaneous nerve, and the supinator muscle, which is innervated by the radial nerve.

10.800–801

What nerve innervates the pronator muscles?

The primary pronators of the forearm are the pronator quadratus and pronator teres, which are both innervated by the median nerve.

10.800–801

What nerve innervates the muscles of the thenar eminence?

The median nerve innervates all the muscles of the thenar eminence except the adductor pollicis brevis, which is innervated by the ulnar nerve.

10.770

What nerve innervates the muscles of the hypothenar eminence and the interossei?

The muscles of the hypothenar eminence and the interossei are innervated by the ulnar nerve.

10.770

What is the significance of having a carrying angle >15° at the elbow and the forearm?

A carrying angle greater than 15° is called cubitus valgus and is significant for abduction of the ulna if somatic dysfunction is present.

6.421

What is the significance of having a carrying angle <3° at the elbow and the forearm?

A carrying angle less than 3° is called cubitus varus and is significant for adduction of the ulna if somatic dysfunction is present.

6.421

In what direction does the radial head move when the forearm is pronated?

The radial head will glide posteriorly when the forearm is pronated.

6.424

In what direction does the radial head move when the forearm is supinated?

The radial head will glide anteriorly when the forearm is supinated.

6.424

What injury causes a posterior radial head?

Most posterior radial head injuries are caused by falling forward on a pronated forearm.

6.424

What injury causes an anterior radial head?

Most anterior radial head injuries are caused by falling backward onto a supinated forearm.

6.424

What is carpal tunnel syndrome?	Carpal tunnel syndrome is entrapment of the median nerve at the flexor retinaculum of the wrist.	10.774
What are the most common symptoms manifested by patients with carpal tunnel syndrome?	Patients with carpal tunnel syndrome complain of paresthesias on the thumb and the first two and one-half digits. In addition, patients also have weakness and atrophy of the ulnar muscles.	10.774
What physical tests are used to diagnose carpal tunnel syndrome?	The Tinel, the Phalen, and the prayer tests are used to diagnose carpal tunnel syndrome.	6.431
What are the gold standard tests for diagnosing carpal tunnel syndrome?	The gold standard tests for diagnosing carpal tunnel syndrome are nerve conduction studies and electromyography.	6.465
What are the osteopathic treatment considerations for carpal tunnel syndrome?	Osteopathic treatment considerations for carpal tunnel syndrome involve treating the rib and upper thoracic somatic dysfunctions to decrease sympathetic tone in the upper extremity and treating cervical somatic dysfunctions and myofascial restrictions to enhance brachial plexus function.	6.465
What is tennis elbow?	Tennis elbow is a strain of the extensor muscles of the forearm of the lateral epicondyle.	6.467
What is the cause of tennis elbow?	Tennis elbow is caused by overuse of the forearm extensors and supinators.	6.467
How is tennis elbow treated?	Tennis elbow is treated using NSAIDs, rest, ice, and OMT.	6.467

What is medial epicondylitis (golfer's elbow)?	Medial epicondylitis is a strain of the flexor muscles of the forearm near the medial epicondyle.	10.746
What is the pathogenesis of medial epicondylitis?	Medial epicondylitis is caused by overuse of the forearm flexor and pronator muscles.	10.746
What is bicipital tenosynovitis?	Bicipital tenosynovitis is inflammation of the tendon and its sheath of the long head of the biceps brachii muscle.	10.771
What is the cause of bicipital tenosynovitis?	Bicipital tenosynovitis is caused by muscle overuse in addition to wear and tear of the tendon on the bicipital groove.	10.771
What is the purpose of the Apley scratch test?	Apley's scratch test is used to evaluate range of motion for the shoulder joint.	6.490
Using the Apley scratch test, how are abduction and external rotation tested?	To test for abduction and external rotation, ask the patient to reach behind his head and touch the opposite shoulder.	6.490
How is internal rotation and adduction evaluated using the Apley scratch test?	To test for adduction and internal rotation, ask the patient to reach in front of her head and touch the opposite shoulder.	6.490
What is the purpose of a drop arm test?	The drop arm test is used to detect rotator cuff tears.	6.416
How is the drop arm test performed?	The drop arm test is performed by asking the patient to abduct the shoulder to 90° and then slowly lower the arm. A positive test results if the patient cannot smoothly lower the arm.	6.416–417

What is Yerguson test?

Yerguson test is used to determine the stability of the bicep tendon in the bicipital groove and is positive if pain is elicited in the tendon of the long head of the biceps when the patient internally rotates the shoulder of a flexed arm against resistance; a positive test indicates possible bicep tendon dislocation or tendonitis.

For boards: You may also encounter the Speed test, which is also used to assess the bicep tendon in the bicipital groove.

6.416

What is the purpose of the Finkelstein test?

The Finkelstein test is used to test the abductor pollicis longus and extensor pollicis brevis tendons at the wrist and is positive if ulnar deviation of the wrist is not possible due to pain; a positive test indicates possible de Quervain tenosynovitis.

6.465

What is the purpose of the Adson test?

The Adson test is used to diagnose thoracic outlet syndrome and is positive if the radial pulse is diminished or lost; symptoms may be further exacerbated by deep inspiration if the diagnosis is difficult to make.

1.701

What is the cause of a positive Adson test?

Performing the Adson test causes the anterior scalene muscle to raise the first rib, which narrows the thoracic outlet, compressing the subclavian artery, which gives rise to the axillary artery, the brachial artery, and then further divides into the ulnar and radial arteries.

1.701

What is the Allen test used for?

The Allen test is used to assess the adequacy of the blood supply to the hand by the radial and ulnar arteries and is positive if capillary refill does not take place in under two seconds; a positive test indicates diminished perfusion and possible occlusion of the radial or ulnar arteries, depending on which artery was compressed.

7.576

What is the purpose of the hip drop test?

The hip drop test is used to assess the sidebending ability of the lumbar spine and the thoracolumbar junction.

1.741

What does a positive hip drop test indicate?

A positive hip drop test is indicative of a somatic dysfunction in the lumbar or thoracolumbar spine.

1.741

What is the purpose of the straight-leg raising test?

The straight-leg raising test is used to evaluate for sciatic nerve compression and is positive if pain radiates past the knee; a positive test indicates possible lumbar disc herniation or sciatic nerve impingement.

6.482

What is the use of the Trendelenberg test?

The Trendelenberg test is used to assess gluteus medius muscle strength and is positive if the patient's hip drops to the contralateral side of the leg the patient is standing on.

6.480

What condition often results in pelvic shift from midline?

Psoas syndrome often results in a flexion contracture leading to a pelvic shift in the opposite direction of the dysfunctional psoas.

6.539

What is the purpose of the Ober test?	The Ober test is used to assess for a tight tensor fascia lata and iliotibial band and is positive if the abducted leg does not freely return to midline; a positive test indicates possible IT iliotibial band contracture.	6.479
What is the significance of the Thomas test?	The Thomas test evaluates for the possibility of a flexion contracture of the hip, usually of iliopsoas origin, and the test is positive if the affected hip is unable to be fully extended.	6.479
When the hip glides anteriorly, in what direction does the femoral head move?	When the hip glides anteriorly, the head of the femur glides anteriorly with external rotation of the hip.	6,479–483
When the hip glides posteriorly, in what direction does the femoral head move?	When the hip glides posteriorly, the head of the femur glides posteriorly with internal rotation of the hip.	6,479–483
What types of somatic dysfunctions are most likely to cause hip restriction with internal rotation?	Piriformis and iliopsoas spasms	6.479
Which joint is the largest joint in the body?	Tibiofemoral joint	6.484
What is the function of the anterior cruciate ligament (ACL)?	The ACL prevents excessive anterior translation of the tibia on the femur.	6.484–485
What is the function of the posterior cruciate ligament (PCL)?	The PCL prevents excessive posterior translation of the tibia on the femur.	6.485
What is the function of medial collateral ligament?	The medial collateral ligament helps to stabilize the knee.	6.484

In what direction does the fibular head move when the foot is pronated?

The fibular head glides anteriorly when the foot is pronated.

6.486

In what direction does the fibular head move when the foot is supinated?

The fibular head glides posteriorly when the foot is supinated.

6.486

What ankle motions occur when the foot is pronated?

Dorsiflexion, eversion, and abduction of the ankle occur when the foot is pronated.

6.498

What ankle motions occur when the foot is supinated?

Plantar flexion, inversion, and adduction of the ankle occur when the foot is supinated.

6.498

What is coxa vara?

Coxa vara occurs when the angle between the neck and shaft of the femur is less than 120°.

6.488

What is coxa valga?

Coxa valga occurs when the angle between the neck and the shaft of the femur is greater than 135°.

6.488

What nerve lies directly posterior to the proximal fibular head?

The common peroneal (fibular) nerve

10.631

What is the cause of patellofemoral syndrome?

Patellofemoral syndrome is an imbalance of the musculature of the quadriceps (strong vastus lateralis and weak vastus medialis).

10.628

How is patellofemoral syndrome treated?

Patellofemoral syndrome is treated by strengthening the vastus medialis muscle.

10.628

True or False: In patellofemoral syndrome, there is a decrease in the Q angle.

False; in patellofemoral syndrome, there is an increase in the Q angle.

10.628

What occurs to the ligament in a first degree sprain?	In first degree ligamentous sprains, there is **no tear** in the ligament; the ligament retains relatively good tensile strength and has no laxity.	1.543
What occurs to the ligament in a second degree sprain?	Second degree ligamentous sprains result in a **partial tear** of the ligament, with decreased tensile strength and mild to moderate laxity.	1.543–544
What occurs to the ligament in a third degree sprain?	Third degree ligamentous sprains involve **complete tear** of the ligament, resulting in no tensile strength and severe laxity.	1.543–544
How many compartments is the lower leg divided into?	The lower leg has four compartments.	10.579
Name the four compartments of the lower leg.	Anterior, lateral, deep posterior, and superficial posterior	10.579
What compartment is most often affected by compartment syndrome?	The anterior compartment is most often affected by compartment syndrome; the diagnosis should not be missed because immediate surgical release is required to prevent permanent damage to the structures within the compartment.	10.580–581
What are the signs of compartment syndrome?	Pain (out of proportion to physical finding and with passive motion or stretch)	1.813
	Pallor	
	Poikilothermia	
	Paresthesias	
	Pulselessness and late paralysis	

What muscle is most affected by anterior compartment syndrome?

The anterior tibialis muscle

10.580

What ligaments are affected in the terrible triad (O'Donahue's triad)?

The ACL medial collateral ligament, and medial meniscus

10.626

What are the main motions of the tibiotalar joint (talocrural joint)?

The main motions of the tibiotalar joint are plantar flexion and dorsiflexion.

6.486

Is the ankle more stable in dorsiflexion or plantarflexion?

The ankle is most stable in **dorsiflexion.**

6.495

How many types of longitudinal arches are present in the foot?

There are two types of longitudinal arches in the foot: the medial and lateral longitudinal arches.

6.499

What structures make up the medial longitudinal arch?

The medial longitudinal arch is made up of the talus, navicular, cuneiforms, and first to third metatarsals.

6.499

What structures make up the lateral longitudinal arch?

The lateral longitudinal arch is made up of the calcaneus, cuboid, and the fourth and fifth metatarsals.

6.499–500

What structures make up the transverse arch?

The transverse arch is made up of the navicular, cuneiform, and cuboid bones.

6.499–500

What arch is most prone to somatic dysfunction?

The transverse arch is very prone to somatic dysfunction, especially in long-distance runners.

6.499

What ligaments are known as the lateral stabilizers of the ankle?

Anterior talofibular ligament, calcaneofibular ligament, and posterior talofibular ligament

6.486

What ligament is the most commonly injured ligament of the ankle?	The anterior talofibular ligament	6.486
What ligament is involved in a type 1 supination sprain of the ankle?	Type 1 supination sprains involve the anterior talofibular ligament.	1.543–544
What ligaments are involved in a type 2 supination sprain of the ankle?	Type 2 supination sprains involve the anterior talofibular ligament and the calcaneofibular ligament.	1.543–544
What ligaments are involved in a type 3 supination sprain of the ankle?	Type 3 supination sprains involve the anterior talofibular ligament, the calcaneofibular ligament, and the posterior talofibular ligament.	1.543–544
What ligament prevents excessive pronation of the ankle?	Deltoid ligament	1.544
True or False: Excessive pronation of ankle will result in a pure ligamentous injury.	**False;** excessive pronation of the ankle will more likely result in a fracture of the medial malleolus.	6.498–502
What is the function of the spring (calcaneonavicular) ligament?	The function of the spring ligament is to strengthen and support the medial longitudinal arch.	6.499
What structures make up the plantar ligament?	The plantar ligament consists of the spring ligament and plantar aponeurosis (plantar fascia).	6.499
Which muscle is considered the primary flexor of the hip?	The iliopsoas muscle	6.473
What muscle is the major hip extensor?	Gluteus maximus	6.473
What muscles are considered the major knee extensors?	The quadriceps (rectus femoris, vastus lateralis, medialis, and intermedius)	6.485

What muscles are considered the major knee flexors?	The semimembranosus and semi-tendinosus (hamstring) muscles	6.473
How many ligaments hold the femoroacetabular joint (hip joint) in place?	Four ligaments hold the femoroacetabular joint in place.	6.471
Name the ligaments that hold the femoroacetabular joint in place.	1. Iliofemoral ligament 2. Ischiofemoral ligament 3. Pubofemoral ligament 4. Capitis femoris	6.471
Which ligament is attached to the head of the femur?	Capitis femoris	6.471
What ligament divides the greater and lesser sciatic foramens?	Sacrospinous ligament	6.473
What is the purpose of the anterior drawer test?	The anterior drawer test is used to assess ACL function and is positive for a possible tear of the ACL if excessive anterior motion is observed during the test.	6.488
What is the purpose of the posterior drawer test?	The posterior drawer test is used to assess PCL function and is positive for a possible tear of the PCL if excessive posterior motion is observed during the test.	6.489
What is the purpose of the Lachman test?	The Lachman the test is used to assess the stability of the ACL and is positive for a possible ACL tear if excessive anterior glide of the tibia is observed during the test.	6.488
What is the purpose of the McMurray the test?	The McMurray test is used to detect tears in the posterior aspect of the menisci and is positive for meniscal damage if pain is elicited during the test.	6.490

What is the purpose of the patellar-grind test?

The patellar-grind test is used to assess the posterior articular surfaces of the patella and is positive for possible chondromalacia patellae if crepitus of the joint is noted during the test.

6.492

What does a valgus stress placed on the knee test?

Valgus stress tests for medial collateral ligament tears.

6.488

What does a varus stress placed on the knee test?

Varus stress tests for lateral collateral ligament tears.

6.488

What is the purpose of the anterior draw test of the ankle?

The anterior draw test of the ankle is used to assess the medial and lateral ligaments of the ankle and is positive for possible ligamentous damage or tears if excessive anterior glide at the ankle is observed during the test.

6.488

What ligaments are assessed using the anterior draw test of the ankle?

The talofibular ligament, superficial ligament, and deltoid ligament

6.488

What is the cause of hallux valgus?

Hallux valgus is a structural deformity of the big toe resulting from contracture of various periarticular structures of the first metatarsophalangeal joint.

1.800

What is the cause of a bunion?

A bunion is caused by varus deviation of the first metatarsal.

1.800

What are hammer toes often associated with?

Hammer toes are often associated with myofascial trigger points in the dorsal interossei of the foot.

1.801

What is sciatica?

Sciatica describes the condition in which patients have pain along the sensory distribution of the sciatic nerve down the back of the leg.

7.711

Name the two nerves that branch from the sciatic nerve.	The common peroneal and tibial nerves	7.711
A decreased Q angle is associated with which one of the following conditions: bow-legged or knock-knee appearance?	A bow-legged appearance	1.791
What ligament is damaged when a child is lifted by the upper limb while the forearm is pronated?	Annular ligament; this condition is known as "nursemaid's elbow."	10.801
What is plantar fasciitis?	Plantar fasciitis is an inflammation of the plantar fascia on the plantar aspect of the foot.	6.542
At what location does the inflammation usually occur?	The inflammation usually occurs at the insertion of the plantar fascia near the calcaneus.	6.542
What OMT approach is used when treating plantar fasciitis?	OMT is directed at freeing motion of the bones of the foot and stretching hypertonic muscles of the calf and fascia.	6.543
What is a march fracture?	A stress fracture found at the shaft of the second or third metatarsal bones	6.542
What causes pes planus?	Pes planus (flat feet) is a condition in which there is dropping of the medial longitudinal arch.	6.543
How is pes planus treated?	Pes planus is treated by prescribing heel wedges or exercises to strengthen the muscles involved.	6.543
What is Morton neuroma?	Morton neuroma is a fibrotendinous reaction occurring between the heads of the third and fourth metatarsals.	6.542

True or False: In Morton neuroma, pain radiates to the toes.	**True;** pain is neuritic in type and radiates to the toes.	6.542
What casues pes anserine bursitis?	Pes anserine bursitis is caused by trauma to the knee joint.	6.541
Contraction of what muscles makes the pain of a pes anserine bursitis worse?	Contraction of the semitendinous, sartorius, and gracilis muscles	6.541
Where is OMT directed to treat pes anserine bursitis?	OMT is directed to the knee, hip, and pelvic regions.	6.541
What is the most common injury to the ankle?	Acute sprain is the most common ankle injury.	6.541
What is the most common cause of acute ankle sprain?	Inversion stress	6.541
What ligament is stretched by inversion of the foot?	Lateral collateral ligament	6.541
What is the common cause of chronic ankle sprains?	Calcaneal valgus stress	6.541
What is meralgia paresthetica?	Meralgia paresthetica is an inflammation of the lateral cutaneous nerve of the femur, also known as "gun-belt neuropathy."	6.539
What physical findings are found in patients with meralgia paresthetica?	Patients with meralgia paresthetica might have a positive Tinel sign present over the lateral femoral cutaneous nerve, oftentimes with a burning pain noted in the nerve's distribution.	6.539
How is the Spencer technique helpful in preventing adhesive capsulitis?	The Spencer technique helps to prevent loss of motion in the painful shoulders and also to restore motion to the shoulder muscles involved.	6.465

What is Dupuytren contracture?

Dupuytren contracture is contracture of the palmar fascia and nodule formation in the palm.

6.465

How does OMT help patients with Dupuytren contracture?

OMT is aimed toward keeping the palmar fascia as free as possible, lessening the contracture.

6.465

What is the use of OMT in patients with de Quervain syndrome?

OMT is directed at improving motion of the joint, decreasing swelling, and treating tenderpoints.

6.465

Name two of the more common types of injuries to the shoulder girdle.

Separation at the acromioclavicular joint and tear of the rotator cuff muscles

6.465

What is the role of OMT in tendonitis of the shoulder joint?

OMT of all the tenderpoints around the shoulder girdle, especially those associated with the tendon, is helpful in diminishing pain.

6.464

What is the most common cause of fractures in the shoulder girdle?

Falls onto an outstretched arm

6.463

What shoulder girdle joints are most prone to somatic dysfunctions?

The sternoclavicular and acromioclavicular joints

6.466

Chapter 4

The Autonomic Nervous System

What are the two components of the peripheral nervous system (PNS)?

The somatic nervous system (SNS) and the autonomic nervous system (ANS)

1.90

What is the main function of the ANS?

To facilitate the normal rhythm of activity in the visceral organs, accommodating for any external challenge

1.90

What is one distinctive feature of the ANS?

The ANS has a two-step output pathway:

1. Preganglionic neurons located centrally
2. Postganglionic neurons located peripherally

1.90

What is facilitation?

An area of impairment or restriction that develops a lower threshold for irritation and dysfunction when other structures are stimulated

6.30

True or False: Facilitation occurs when more afferent stimulation is needed to trigger a discharge of impulses.

False; in a facilitated state, less afferent stimulation is needed for discharge of impulses because of hypersensitization of afferent fibers.

6.30

List the three components of the spinal reflex.

1. An afferent limb (sensory input)
2. A central limb (spinal pathway)
3. An efferent limb (motor pathway)

6.30

Table 4–1. Sympathetic Innervation

	Cord Level	Ganglion	Nerve
Head and neck	T1-T4		
Heart	T1-T5		
Lungs and respiratory system	T2-T7		
Esophagus	T2-T8		
Upper extremities	T2-T8		
Upper GI tract			
Gallbladder, liver, spleen, stomach	T5-T9	Celiac	Greater splanchnic
Segments of the pancreas and duodenum	T5-T9	Celiac	Greater splanchnic
Middle GI tract			
Segments of the pancreas and duodenum	T10-T11	Superior mesenteric	Lesser splanchnic
Jejunum and ilium	T10-T11	Superior mesenteric	Lesser splanchnic
Ascending colon	T10-T11	Superior mesenteric	Lesser splanchnic
Initial 2/3 of the transverse colon	T10-T11	Superior mesenteric	Lesser splanchnic
Kidneys and upper ureters	T10-T11	Superior mesenteric	
Lower GI tract			
Final 1/3 of the transverse colon	T12-L2	Inferior mesenteric	Least splanchnic
Descending and sigmoid colons	T12-L2	Inferior mesenteric	Least splanchnic
Rectum	T12-L2	Inferior mesenteric	Least splanchnic
Lower ureters	T12-L1	Inferior mesenteric	
Adrenal medulla	T10		
Testes and ovaries	T10-T11		
Uterus and cervix	T10-L2		
Cisterna chyli	T11		
Erectile tissue (penis and clitoris)	T11-L2		

Table 4–1. **Sympathetic Innervation (*Continued*)**

	Cord Level	Ganglion	Nerve
Bladder	T11-L2		
Legs	T11-L2		
Appendix	T12		
Prostate	T12-L2		
Parasympathetic innervation			
Everything above the diaphragm			Vagus nerve
Ascending and transverse colon			Vagus nerve
Kidneys and upper ureters			Vagus nerve
Testes and ovaries			Vagus nerve
All other reproductive organs (not testes and ovaries)			Pelvic splanchnic
Descending and recto-sigmoid colons			Pelvic splanchnic
Lower ureters and bladder			Pelvic splanchnic

List the three areas that can be facilitated.	1. Higher centers (brain) 2. Viscera, via sympathetic or parasympathetic visceral afferents 3. Somatic afferents (muscle spindles, golgi tendons, nociceptors, etc.)	6.30
What is a viscerosomatic reflex?	Localized visceral stimuli producing patterns of reflex response, in segmentally related somatic structures	6.29–30
Give an example of a viscerosomatic reflex.	Acute cholecystitis often refers pain to the midthoracic region at the tip of the right scapula.	1.105– 111, 6.29–30

Give other examples of a viscerosomatic reflex.	T1-T5 somatic dysfunction, and pain radiating into the jaw and left arm associated with cardiac abnormalities, such as a myocardial infarction	1.105–111, 6.29–30
What is a somatovisceral reflex?	Somatic stimuli producing patterns of reflex response in segmentally related visceral structures.	1.1048–1049
Give an example of a somatovisceral reflex.	A trigger point is located in the right pectoralis major muscle, between the fifth and sixth ribs and just medial to the nipple line, that has been known to cause supraventricular tachyarrhythmias.	1.1048–1049
What effect does the parasympathetic nervous system have on the pupils of the eyes?	It causes constriction of the pupils, also known as *miosis*.	1.99–100
What effect does the parasympathetic nervous system have on the lenses of the eyes?	It causes the lenses to contract for near vision, also known as *accommodation*.	1.99–100
What effect does the parasympathetic nervous system have on the glands (nasal, lacrimal, parotid, submandibular, gastric, and pancreatic) of the body?	It stimulates these glands to secrete their products.	1.99–100
What effect does the parasympathetic nervous system have on the sweat glands?	It stimulates the palms of the hands to sweat.	1.98–99
What effect does the parasympathetic nervous system have on the heart?	It decreases contractility (inotropy) and conduction velocity.	1.101–102

What effect does the parasympathetic nervous system have on the bronchiolar smooth muscle of the lungs?	It causes contraction of the bronchiolar smooth muscle of the lungs.	1.102–103
What effect does the parasympathetic nervous system have on the respiratory epithelium of the lungs?	It decreases the number of goblet cells and thins secretions.	1.102–103
What effect does the parasympathetic nervous system have on the smooth muscle lumen of the gastrointestinal (GI) tract?	It causes contraction of the lumen of the GI tract.	1.104–111
What effect does the parasympathetic nervous system have on the smooth muscle sphincters within the GI tract?	It causes relaxation of the sphincters within the GI tract.	1.104–111
What effect does the parasympathetic nervous system have on secretion and motility within the GI tract?	It increases the amount of secretion and motility within the GI tract.	1.104–111
What effect does the parasympathetic nervous system have on the skin and visceral vessels?	The parasympathetic nervous system has **no effect** on the skin and visceral vessels.	1.97–98
What effect does the parasympathetic nervous system have on skeletal muscle?	The parasympathetic nervous system has **no effect** on skeletal muscle.	1.97–98
What effect does the parasympathetic nervous system have on the bladder wall (detrusor muscle)?	It causes contraction of the bladder wall.	1.113–114

What effect does the parasympathetic nervous system have on the bladder sphincter (trigone)?	It causes relaxation of the bladder sphincter.	1.113–114
What is the parasympathetic nervous system function on the penis?	It causes erection of the penis. *Note:* A good way to remember this is to think "point & shoot." Point is the erection portion controlled by the PNS; shoot is the ejaculation portion controlled by the SNS.	1.116
What effect does the parasympathetic nervous system have on the kidneys?	The effect of the parasympathetic nervous system on the kidneys is unknown.	1.111–112
What effect does the parasympathetic nervous system have on the ureters?	It maintains normal peristalsis.	1.112–113
What effect does the parasympathetic nervous system have on the liver?	It causes slight glycogen synthesis.	1.111
What effect does the parasympathetic nervous system have on the body (fundus) of the uterus?	It causes relaxation of the body (fundus) of the uterus.	1.115–116
What effect does the parasympathetic nervous system have on the cervix of the uterus?	It causes constriction of the cervix of the uterus.	1.115–116
What effect does the sympathetic nervous system have on the pupils of the eyes?	It causes dilation of the pupils, also known as *mydriasis.*	1.99–100
What effect does the sympathetic nervous system have on the lenses of the eyes?	It causes lenses of the eyes to slightly relax to allow for better far vision.	1.99–100

What effect does the sympathetic nervous system have on the glands (nasal, lacrimal, parotid, submandibular, gastric, and pancreatic) of the body?	It causes vasoconstriction of these glands for slight secretion of their products.	1.99–100
What effect does the sympathetic nervous system have on the sweat glands?	It causes heavy sweating.	1.98–99
What effect does the sympathetic nervous system have on the heart?	It increases contractility (inotropy) and conduction velocity.	1.101–102
What effect does the sympathetic nervous system have on the bronchiolar smooth muscle of the lungs?	It relaxes the bronchiolar smooth muscle of the lungs.	1.102–103
What effect does the sympathetic nervous system have on the respiratory epithelium of the lungs?	It increases the number of goblet cells to produce thick secretions.	1.102–103
What effect does the sympathetic nervous system have on the smooth muscle lumen within the GI tract?	It causes relaxation of the smooth muscle lumen within the GI tract.	1.104–111
What effect does the sympathetic nervous system have on the smooth muscle sphincters within the GI tract?	It causes contraction of the smooth muscle sphincters within the GI tract.	1.104–111
What effect does the sympathetic nervous system have on the secretions and motility within the GI tract?	It decreases the secretions and motility within the GI tract.	1.104–111
What effect does the sympathetic nervous system have on the skin and visceral vessels?	It causes contraction of the skin and visceral vessels.	1.97–98

What effect does the sympathetic nervous system have on skeletal muscle?	It causes relaxation of skeletal muscle.	1.97–98
What effect does the sympathetic nervous system have on the bladder wall (detrusor)?	It causes relaxation of the bladder wall (detrusor).	1.113–114
What effect does the sympathetic nervous system have on the bladder sphincter (trigone)?	It causes contraction of the bladder sphincter (trigone).	1.113–114
What effect does the sympathetic nervous system have on the penis?	It causes ejaculation.	1.116
What effect does the sympathetic nervous system have on the kidneys?	It causes vasoconstriction of afferent arterioles, which decreases the glomerular filtration rate and results in decreased urine volume.	1.111–112
What effect does the sympathetic nervous system have on the ureters?	It causes ureterospasm.	1.112–113
What effect does the sympathetic nervous system have on the liver?	It causes glycogenolysis, which increases the release of glucose into the bloodstream.	1.111
What effect does the sympathetic nervous system have on the body (fundus) of the uterus?	It causes constriction of the body (fundus) of the uterus.	1.115–116
What effect does the sympathetic nervous system have on the cervix of the uterus?	It causes relaxation of the uterine cervix.	1.115–116
From where does cranial nerve CN III emerge?	CN III emerges from the midbrain.	5.654–655

Which ganglion within the parasympathetic nervous system causes constriction of the pupils?	The ciliary ganglion	5.654–655
From were does CN VII emerge?	CN VII emerges from the pontomedullary junction.	5.658–660
Name the two ganglions involved in parasympathetic nervous system activity that are located within CN VII.	Pterygopalatine ganglion and submandibular ganglion	5.660
Within the parasympathetic nervous system, what glands are associated with the pterygopalatine ganglion?	The lacrimal glands	5.660
Within the parasympathetic nervous system, what glands are associated with the submandibular ganglion?	The submandibular and sublingual glands	5.660
From where does CN IX emerge?	CN IX emerges from the medulla of the brain.	5.662–663
What ganglion involved in parasympathetic nervous system activity is controlled by CN IX?	The otic ganglion	5.662–663
What glands are parasympathetically associated with the otic ganglion?	The parotid glands	5.663
From where does CN X emerge?	CN X emerges as a series of rootlets on the side of the medulla.	5.664–666
What effect does CN X have on the heart?	It decreases contractility and conduction velocity.	1.101–102

What effect does CN X have on the lungs?	It causes contraction of the bronchiolar smooth muscle and decreases the number of goblet cells to enhance thin secretions within the respiratory epithelium.	1.102–103
What CN innervates the lower two-thirds of the esophagus?	CN X (the vagus nerve)	1.104–111
What CN innervates the stomach?	CN X (the vagus nerve)	1.104–111
What CN innervates the small intestine?	CN X (the vagus nerve)	1.104–111
What CN innervates the liver?	CN X (the vagus nerve)	1.104–111
What CN innervates the gallbladder?	CN X (the vagus nerve)	1.104–111
What CN innervates the pancreas?	CN X (the vagus nerve)	1.104–111
What two organs of the urinary system are parasympathetically innervated by CN X?	The kidneys and upper ureters	1.111–113
What two organs of the reproductive system are parasympathetically innervated by CN X?	The testes and ovaries	1.114–116
What two organs of the GI system are parasympathetically innervated by CN X?	The ascending colon and transverse colon	1.104–111
What spinal cord levels make up the pelvic splanchnic nerve?	The S2-S4 spinal cord levels	1.113–116

What two organs of the urinary system are parasympathetically innervated by the pelvic splanchnic nerve?	The lower ureters and bladder	1.112–114
What female organ of the reproductive system is parasympathetically innervated by the pelvic splanchnic nerve?	The uterus	1.114–116
What male organ of the reproductive system is parasympathetically innervated by the pelvic splanchnic nerve?	The prostate	1.114–116
What organ of the reproductive system is parasympathetically innervated by the pelvic splanchnic nerve?	The genitalia	1.114–116
What three organs of the GI system are parasympathetically innervated by the pelvic splanchnic nerve?	The descending colon, sigmoid colon, and rectum	1.104–111
True or False: Segmental sympathetic innervation levels are the same in every individual.	**False;** the innervation levels vary from individual to individual. *Note:* It is important to be familiar with innervation levels, but keep in mind that these levels vary in each individual; as with all aspects of medicine, clinical judgment should be heavily relied upon by the experienced physician.	1.94–96
What spinal cord levels sympathetically innervate the head and neck?	The T1-T4 spinal cord levels	1.99–100

What spinal cord levels sympathetically innervate the heart?	The T1-T5 spinal cord levels	1.101–102
What spinal cord levels sympathetically innervate the respiratory system?	The T2-T7 spinal cord levels	1.103
What spinal cord levels sympathetically innervate the esophagus?	The T2-T8 spinal cord levels	1.103–104
Which organs are considered part of the upper GI tract?	1. Gallbladder 2. Liver 3. Stomach 4. Spleen 5. Proximal duodenum 6. Portions of pancreas	1.106
From which portion of the embryological gut did the organs of the upper GI tract originate?	The foregut	1.106
Which organs are considered part of the middle GI tract?	1. Distal duodenum 2. Portions of pancreas 3. Jejunum 4. Ilium 5. Ascending colon 6. Proximal two-thirds of transverse colon	1.107
From which portion of the embryological gut did the organs of the middle GI tract originate?	The midgut	1.107
Which organs are considered part of the lower GI tract?	1. Distal one-third of transverse colon 2. Descending colon 3. Sigmoid colon 4. Rectum	1.107–111

From which portion of the embryological gut did the organs of the lower GI tract originate?	The hindgut	1.109–111
What spinal cord levels sympathetically innervate the stomach?	The T5-T9 spinal cord levels	5.45
What spinal cord levels sympathetically innervate the liver?	The T5-T9 spinal cord levels	5.45
What spinal cord levels sympathetically innervate the gallbladder?	The T5-T9 spinal cord levels	5.45
What spinal cord levels sympathetically innervate the spleen?	The T5-T9 spinal cord levels	5.45
What spinal cord levels sympathetically innervate the proximal duodenum and portions of the pancreas?	The T5-T9 spinal cord levels	1.105–111
What corresponding nerve sympathetically innervates the stomach?	The greater splanchnic nerve	5.45
What corresponding nerve sympathetically innervates the liver?	The greater splanchnic nerve	5.45
What corresponding nerve sympathetically innervates the gallbladder?	The greater splanchnic nerve	5.45
What corresponding nerve sympathetically innervates the spleen?	The greater splanchnic nerve	5.45
What corresponding nerve sympathetically innervates the proximal duodenum and portions of the pancreas?	The greater splanchnic nerve	1.105–111

What corresponding ganglion sympathetically innervates the stomach?	The celiac ganglion	1.106
What corresponding ganglion sympathetically innervates the liver?	The celiac ganglion	1.106
What corresponding ganglion sympathetically innervates the gallbladder?	The celiac ganglion	1.106
What corresponding ganglion sympathetically innervates the spleen?	The celiac ganglion	1.106
What corresponding ganglion sympathetically innervates the proximal duodenum and portions of the pancreas?	The celiac ganglion	1.106
What spinal cord levels sympathetically innervate the distal duodenum and portions of the pancreas?	The T10-T11 spinal cord levels	1.107–111
What spinal cord levels sympathetically innervate the jejunum?	The T10-T11 spinal cord levels	1.107–111
What spinal cord levels sympathetically innervate the ilium?	The T10-T11 spinal cord levels	1.107–111
What spinal cord levels sympathetically innervate the ascending colon?	The T10-T11 spinal cord levels	1.107–111
What spinal cord levels sympathetically innervate the proximal two-thirds of the transverse colon?	The T10-T11 spinal cord levels	1.107–111

What corresponding nerve sympathetically innervates the distal duodenum and portions of the pancreas?	The lesser splanchnic nerve	1.107– 111
What corresponding nerve sympathetically innervates the jejunum?	The lesser splanchnic nerve	1.107– 111
What corresponding nerve sympathetically innervates the ilium?	The lesser splanchnic nerve	1.107– 111
What corresponding nerve sympathetically innervates the ascending colon?	The lesser splanchnic nerve	1.107– 111
What corresponding nerve sympathetically innervates the proximal two-thirds of transverse colon?	The lesser splanchnic nerve	1.107– 111
What corresponding ganglion sympathetically innervates the distal duodenum and portions of the pancreas?	The superior mesenteric ganglion	1.107
What corresponding ganglion sympathetically innervates the jejunum?	The superior mesenteric ganglion	1.107
What corresponding ganglion sympathetically innervates the ilium?	The superior mesenteric ganglion	1.107
What corresponding ganglion sympathetically innervates the ascending colon?	The superior mesenteric ganglion	1.107
What corresponding ganglion sympathetically innervates the proximal two-thirds of the transverse colon?	The superior mesenteric ganglion	1.107

What spinal cord levels sympathetically innervate the distal one-third of the transverse colon?	The T12-L2 spinal cord levels	1.107–111
What spinal cord levels sympathetically innervate the descending colon?	The T12-L2 spinal cord levels	1.107–111
What spinal cord levels sympathetically innervate the sigmoid colon?	The T12-L2 spinal cord levels	1.107–111
What spinal cord levels sympathetically innervate the rectum?	The T12-L2 spinal cord levels	1.107–111
What corresponding nerve sympathetically innervates the distal one-third of the transverse colon?	The least splanchnic nerve	1.107–111
What corresponding nerve sympathetically innervates the descending colon?	The least splanchnic nerve	1.107–111
What corresponding nerve sympathetically innervates the sigmoid colon?	The least splanchnic nerve	1.107–111
What corresponding nerve sympathetically innervates the rectum?	The least splanchnic nerve	1.107–111
What corresponding ganglion sympathetically innervates the distal one-third of the transverse colon?	The inferior mesenteric ganglion	1.107–111
What corresponding ganglion sympathetically innervates the descending colon?	The inferior mesenteric ganglion	1.107–111

What corresponding ganglion sympathetically innervates the sigmoid colon?	The inferior mesenteric ganglion	1.107–111
What corresponding ganglion sympathetically innervates the rectum?	The inferior mesenteric ganglion	1.107–111
What spinal cord level sympathetically innervates the appendix?	The T10 spinal cord level	5.161
What spinal cord levels sympathetically innervate the kidneys?	The T10-T11 spinal cord levels	1.111–112
What corresponding ganglion sympathetically innervates the kidneys?	The superior mesenteric ganglion	1.111–112
What spinal cord level sympathetically innervates the adrenals?	The T10 spinal cord level	1.111–112
What spinal cord levels sympathetically innervate the upper ureters?	The T10-T11 spinal cord levels	1.112–113
What corresponding ganglion sympathetically innervates the upper ureters?	The superior mesenteric ganglion	1.112–113
What spinal cord levels sympathetically innervate the lower ureters?	The T12-L1 spinal cord levels	1.112–113
What corresponding ganglion sympathetically innervates the lower ureters?	The inferior mesenteric ganglion	1.112–113
What spinal cord levels sympathetically innervate the bladder?	The T11-L2 spinal cord levels	1.113–114

What spinal cord levels sympathetically innervate the gonads?	The T10-T11 spinal cord levels	1.114–115
What spinal cord levels sympathetically innervate the uterus?	The T10-L2 spinal cord levels	1.114–116
What spinal cord levels sympathetically innervate the uterus?	The T10-L2 spinal cord levels	1.114–116
What spinal cord levels sympathetically innervate the erectile tissue of the penis?	The T11-L2 spinal cord levels	1.116
What spinal cord levels sympathetically innervate the erectile tissue of the clitoris?	The T11-L2 spinal cord levels	1.116
What spinal cord levels sympathetically innervate the prostate?	The T12-L2 spinal cord levels	1.114–115
What spinal cord levels sympathetically innervate the upper extremities (arms)?	The T2-T8 spinal cord levels	1.97–98
What spinal cord levels sympathetically innervate the lower extremities (legs)?	The T11-L2 spinal cord levels	1.97–98
Name the three main organ systems below the diaphragm.	The GI system, the genitourinary (GU) system, and the reproductive system	
The entire small intestine is innervated by what nerve of the parasympathetic nervous system?	CN X (the vagus nerve)	5.153–160
What are the names of the four segments into which the colon is divided?	The ascending, transverse, descending, and rectosigmoid segments	5.160–164

What two segments are considered the proximal half of the large intestine?	The ascending colon and the transverse colon	5.160–164
What two segments are considered the distal half of the large intestine?	The descending colon and the rectosigmoid colon	5.160–164
The proximal half of the large intestine is parasympathetically innervated by what CN?	CN X (the vagus nerve)	5.153–160, 1.111–114
The distal half of the large intestine is parasympathetically innervated by what nerve?	The pelvic splanchnic nerve	5.153–160, 1.111–114
What are the three major organ systems of the GU system?	The kidneys, ureters (upper and lower), and bladder	5.180–185, 1.111–114
What two sections are considered the proximal half of the GU system?	The kidneys and upper ureters	5.180–185, 1.111–114
What two sections are considered the distal half of the GU system?	The lower ureters and bladder	5.180–185, 1.111–114
The proximal half of the GU system is parasympathetically innervated by what CN?	CN X (the vagus nerve)	5.180–185, 1.111–114
The distal half of the GU system is parasympathetically innervated by what nerve?	The pelvic splanchnic nerve	5.180–185, 1.111–114
True or False: All reproductive structures are parasympathetically innervated by the pelvic splanchnic nerve.	**False;** all reproductive structures except the ovaries and testes are innervated by the pelvic splanchnic nerve. *Note:* The ovaries and testes are innervated by the vagus nerve.	1.114–116

What significance does the ligament of Treitz hold as a landmark?	It divides the duodenum and jejunum.	5.153–156
What significance does the splenic flexure of the large intestine hold as a landmark?	It divides the transverse and descending colon.	5.161–164
What spinal cord levels sympathetically innervate the organs before the ligament of Treitz?	The T5-T9 spinal cord levels	1.106–117
What spinal cord levels sympathetically innervate the organs between the ligament of Treitz and splenic flexure?	The T10-T11 spinal cord levels	1.106–17
What spinal cord levels sympathetically innervate the visceral organs past the splenic flexure?	The T12-L2 spinal cord levels	1.106–117

Chapter 5 — **Lymphatics**

What are the main functions of the lymphatic system?	1. Maintaining fluid balance 2. Purification and cleansing of tissues 3. Defense against toxins, bacteria, and viruses 4. Nutrition	1.1059
Into which lymphatic duct do the right side of the head and neck, the right upper extremity, and the right half of the thoracic cavity drain?	The right lymphatic duct	9.36–38
The remainder (most) of the body drains into which lymphatic duct?	The left lymphatic (thoracic) duct	9.37–38
Where does the right lymphatic duct drain into?	The right brachiocephalic vein	1.1058
Where does the left lymphatic duct drain into?	The junction of the left internal jugular and subclavian veins	9.36
What effect does the sympathetic nervous system have on lymphatics?	It constricts the lymphatic vessels.	1.1064
What are the results of constricting the lymphatic vessels?	Initially, there is an increase in lymph peristalsis; however, sustained hypersympathetic tone will decrease lymphatic movement.	1.1064
What effect does osteopathic manipulative therapy (OMT) and exercise have on lymphatic fluid movement?	It increases lymphatic fluid circulation.	1.1060

True or False: Decreased interstitial fluid pressure will increase lymphatic fluid movement.

False; any increase in interstitial fluid pressure will increase the absorption of lymph into lymph capillaries.

1.1060

True or False: Contraction of the diaphragm and other muscles of the body decreases lymphatic fluid movement.

False; muscle contraction will increase movement of lymphatic fluid.

6.587, 1.1060

True or False: Restricted thoracic cage motion or a tense pelvic diaphragm can lead to lymphatic congestion.

True; any restriction within the body has the potential to cause lymphatic congestion.

6.587

What lymphatic treatment increases total body lymphatic movement and is useful for pediatric patients?

The Dalrymple pedal pump

1.1062

Which lymphatic treatment increases rib cage motion in addition to increasing total body lymphatic movement?

The Miller lymphatic (thoracic) pump

1.1068

Which treatment techniques can decrease dural strains and increase venous return from the head?

Cranial techniques

1.1065

What lymphatic treatment technique will increase thoracic motion by decreasing somatic dysfunction of the ribs, spine, and sternomanubrial-clavicular complex?

Rib raising

1.1062, 1.1064

What treatment technique will normalize hypersympa-thetic activity and mobilize the ribs for improved respiration?

Rib raising

1.1062, 1.1064

True or False: An anterior cervical fascia release will encourage lymphatic drainage.

True; any release of restrictions throughout the body has the potential to encourage lymphatic drainage.

1.1072

What treatment consists of wave like motions of the arms and legs to help direct lymph movement out of an area of congestion?

The treatment technique known as *effleurage*

1.1076

What treatment facilitates the movement of toxins and other antigens to liver macrophages (Kupffer cells) and encourages screening and removal of damaged cells by the spleen?

The liver (splenic) pump

1.1070

What technique uses stroking of the skin overlying the mandible to force fluids through congested lymphatic vessels and has been shown to improve and shorten the expected course of patients with otitis media?

The Galbraith technique

1.1071,
1.1241

What treatment technique should be used first when treating a dysfunction of lymphatic drainage?

Treatment of the thoracic inlet should be used first when treating a dysfunction of lymphatic drainage because it is the space where most of the lymphatic fluid eventually drains back into the venous circulation; if it is congested, all other lymphatic channels will be adversely affected.

1.1062–
1063

What treatment is recommended second, after treating the thoracic inlet?

Rib raising

1.1062

What is the third step in the treatment of lymphatic dysfunction?

Redoming the thoracoabdominal diaphragm

1.1062

What treatment will optimize thoracoabdominal pressure gradients, thereby maximizing lymph return?

Redoming the thoracoabdominal diaphragm

1.1062

At what point should lymphatic pump techniques be used to treat lymphatic dysfunctions?

Lymphatic pump techniques should be used after treatment of the thoracic inlet, rib raising, and redoming of the thoracoabdominal diaphragm.

1.1062

What are the relative contraindications for lymphatic treatment?

1. Carcinoma
2. Bone fractures in the area of treatment
3. Abscess or localized infection
4. Bacterial infection with temperature >102°F

1.1062, 6.591

Chapter 6

Articulatory Techniques and Myofascial Release

Are articulatory techniques considered direct or indirect?	Articulatory techniques are gentle **direct** techniques that are used to increase range of motion in a restricted joint.	1.834
What types of patients are most likely to respond to articulatory techniques?	Elderly patients and postoperative patients, because the techniques are gentle in nature	1.835
What are the indications for articulatory techniques?	1. The patient must have limited or lost articular motion. 2. To normalize sympathetic tone. 3. To increase the frequency and amplitude of a joint's range of motion.	1.836
What are the contraindications for articulatory techniques?	Articulatory techniques are not used in patients with acutely inflamed joints and fractures. Also, avoid using these types of techniques in the cervical region because of the possibility of vertebral artery compression.	1.835–837
What are the two most frequently used articulatory techniques?	The Spencer technique and rib raising	1.836–837
What is the purpose of the Spencer technique?	The purpose of the Spencer technique is to improve motion in the glenohumeral joint, thereby increasing range of motion.	1.836

How many stages are there in the Spencer technique?

There are seven stages in the Spencer technique.

1.836

What is stage I of the Spencer technique?

Stage I involves stretching the tissues and pumping fluid with the arm extended.

1.836

What is stage II of the Spencer technique?

Stage II involves glenohumeral flexion/extension with the elbow flexed.

1.836

What is stage III of the Spencer technique?

Stage III involves glenohumeral flexion/extension with the elbow extended.

1.836

What is stage IV of the Spencer technique?

Stage IV involves circumduction with both compression and traction, repeating the technique with the arm both flexed and extended.

1.836

What is stage V of the Spencer technique?

Stage V involves adduction and external rotation with the elbow flexed.

1.836

What is stage VI of the Spencer technique?

Stage VI involves abduction and internal rotation with the arm behind the back.

1.836

What is the seventh and final stage of the Spencer technique?

Stage VII involves stretching tissues and pumping fluids with the arm extended.

1.836

What musculoskeletal condition is a Spencer technique useful for?

The Spencer technique is useful in treating patients with adhesive capsulitis.

6.444

What is the purpose of rib raising?

The purpose of rib raising is to increase chest wall motion, improve lymphatic return, and normalize sympathetic tone.

1.835

Patients with what respiratory illness are most likely to benefit from rib raising?	Patients with pneumonia are most likely to benefit from this technique because it increases lymphatic flow.	1.835
True or False: Rib raising reduces sympathetic activity.	**True;** rib raising is used to decrease and thereby normalize sympathetic activity.	1.835
What is the myofascial release technique?	Myofascial release is a technique that combines several types of osteopathic manipulative therapy (OMT) in order to stretch and release muscle and fascial restrictions.	1.1158
What are the goals of myofascial release treatment?	To restore functional balance to all tissues and improve lymphatic flow	1.1158
What are the indications for myofascial release treatment?	Myofascial release can be performed on acutely ill patients and elderly patients who cannot tolerate aggressive therapy.	1.1158
What is the difference between the right and left lymphatic drainage of the upper extremities?	The right lymphatic duct drains the right upper extremity, including the left lower lobe of the lung and the heart; the left lymphatic drains the left upper extremity and the rest of the body.	8.324
True or False: The left lymphatic duct is the minor duct, and the right lymphatic duct is the major duct.	**False;** the right lymphatic duct is referred to as the minor duct, and the left lymphatic duct is referred to as the major duct.	8.324
Is myofascial release passive or active, direct or indirect?	Myofascial release can be passive or active, direct or indirect.	1.836

What are the steps in performing the myofascial release procedure?

1. Palpate the restriction.   1.836
2. Apply compression (indirect) or traction (direct).
3. Add twisting or transverse forces.
4. Use enhancers such as respiration, eye movement, and muscle contraction.
5. Feel for and await the release.

What are the contraindications for myofascial release?

Fractures in the area being treated and lymphatic system malignancies   1.836

What is the purpose of myofascial release?

To improve lymphatic flow to all tissues by removing myofascial restrictions   1.836

Chapter 7　Counterstrain

Is counterstrain a direct or indirect treatment?	Counterstrain is an indirect treatment technique.	1.1002
What is the first step in using counterstrain as a treatment?	Finding a significant tenderpoint	1.1003–1004
What is the goal of counterstrain?	To normalize the gamma efferent system to facilitate the removal of somatic dysfunction	1.1003
What is a tenderpoint?	A small, tense area the size of a fingertip that is extremely tender to palpation	1.1004
Where are tenderpoints usually located?	Tendinous attachments, the belly of a muscle, and other myofascial tissues such as ligaments	1.1004
If there are multiple tenderpoints in a certain area, which tenderpoint do you treat first?	The most severe (sensitive) tenderpoint	1.1004–1005
After finding the tenderpoint, what is the next treatment step?	To place the patient into a position of ease	1.1004–1005
If several tenderpoints of equal tenderness occur in a row, which one is treated first?	The middle tenderpoint is treated first.	1.1007
When is the optimal position of comfort obtained?	The optimal position of comfort is obtained when palpation of the tenderpoint no longer elicits discomfort. For boards, know that a physician needs to reduce the tenderness by 70%.	1.1007

How is the level of discomfort associated with a tenderpoint monitored?

On a 0 to 10 scale, with 10 being the most severe

1.1005

Do tenderpoints radiate pain?

No; tenderpoints do not radiate pain; however, trigger points do.

1.1003–1005, 1.1035–1038

How long should a position of comfort be maintained when treating a tenderpoint using counterstrain?

A position of comfort should be maintained for 90 seconds.

1.1006

True or False: As you position the patient in ease, you want to reduce the tenderness of a tenderpoint by at least 30%.

False; you want to reduce the tenderness at least 70% (3 out of 10 on a subjective pain scale with 10 being the worst pain a person has ever felt).

1.1006–1007

What are some common mistakes physicians make when using counterstrain that can cause the treatment to be ineffective?

1. The patient is moved back to neutral too quickly.
2. The patient or the physician is not relaxed.
3. The patient is not optimally positioned.
4. The most significant tenderpoint is not treated.

1.1006

When is treatment with counterstrain considered successful?

When no more than 30% of the original tenderness remains

1.1007

What is the last step in a counterstrain treatment?

Recheck the tenderpoint

Note: For practical purposes, always recheck your somatic findings after any osteopathic therapy.

1.1004

True or False: For maximum results, the patient must be completely relaxed during treatment.

True; any tension on the part of the patient has the potential to hamper the treatment results.

1.1007

Are there any complications or side effects associated with counterstrain?	**Yes;** a generalized soreness or flu-like reaction is sometimes observed.	1.1006–1007
Does this reaction occur in all patients?	**No;** it occurs in approximately 30% of patients.	1.1007
When does this reaction occur?	Within the first 48 hours after treatment	1.1007
Is there anything that can be prescribed to help reduce this reaction?	Analgesics for 1 to 2 days following treatment with counterstrain	1.1007
What is a therapeutic pulse?	A pulsation felt by the physician when treating the tenderpoint	1.1003
When is the therapeutic pulse felt?	It only occurs when the patient is moved close to the position of comfort.	1.1003
How long is the pulse felt?	It disappears after myofascial tissue relaxation.	1.1003
How long does it take for myofascial tissue relaxation to occur?	90 seconds	1.1003
Is the therapeutic pulse felt with every tenderpoint?	**No;** it does not occur with every tenderpoint.	1.1003
What is the therapeutic pulse associated with?	Improved treatment response	1.1003–1004
True or False: In general, the typical treatment position for anterior tenderpoints is flexion.	**True;** as a general rule, most anterior tenderpoints are treated in the flexion position.	1.1007
How can counterstrain treatments be easily remembered for practical application?	The goal of any counterstrain techniques is to "curl" the patient's surrounding muscle groups around the point of	

treatment. For example, counterstrain of the biceps muscle would involve flexing and supinating the biceps muscle around the counterstrain point.

In general, what is the typical treatment position for posterior tenderpoints?

Positioning the patient in *extension*

1.1007

What treatment positions are typically used for tenderpoints more lateral to the midline?

More rotation and sidebending

1.1006–1007

True or False: Midline tenderpoints typically require pure flexion (if anterior) or pure extension (if posterior).

This is generally true.

1.1006–1007

While maintaining contact with the tenderpoint, the physician should be monitoring for what kinds of change?

Myofascial changes such as ease in tissue tension and a reduction in tenderpoint discomfort

1.1006–1007

What is a Maverick point?

Tenderpoints that are treated by positioning the patient opposite of what is typically expected

1.1007

Which region of the body has the most Maverick points?

The cervical spine

1.1007

Within the cervical spine, where are the anterior tenderpoints typically located?

At the lateral aspect of the lateral masses or anterior to the lateral masses

1.1007–1008

Where are the posterior tenderpoints in the cervical spine typically located?

1. On the occiput
2. Tip of the spinous processes or just lateral to the spinous processes

1.1007–1008

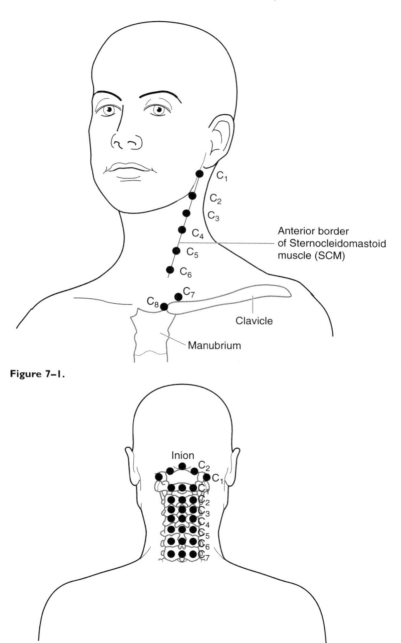

Figure 7–1.

Figure 7–2.

Where is the tenderpoint for the anterior first cervical located?	At the posterior edge of the ascending ramus of the mandible at the lobe of the ear	1.1007
What is the counterstrain treatment position for the anterior first cervical?	Rotation of the head about 90° away from the tenderpoint	1.1007
Where are the tenderpoints for anterior levels C2-C6 located?	At the anterior surface on the transverse processes of the corresponding vertebrae	1.1007–1008
What is the treatment position for anterior C2-C6?	**FS$_A$R$_A$** (**F**lex the head and neck to 45°; **S**idebend **A**way and **R**otate the head **A**way from the tenderpoint)	1.1008
Where are the tenderpoints for anterior levels C7 and C8 located?	Anterior C7: 2 to 3 cm lateral to the medial end of the clavicle Anterior C8: the medial end of the clavicle at the sternal notch	1.1008
What are the treatment positions for anterior C7 and C8?	C7: Flexion, sidebend toward and rotate away from tenderpoint C8: Flexion, sidebend away and rotate away (**FS$_A$R$_A$**)	1.1007–1008, 11.43–44
Where are the tenderpoints for posterior cervical levels C2-C7 located?	At the tips of the spinous process	1.1008
True or False: The treatment position for posterior cervical C2-C7 tenderpoints is extension, rotation away, and sidebending away from the side of the tenderpoint.	**False;** C2 and C4-C7 are extension, sidebending away, and rotation away (ES$_A$R$_A$). C3 is flexion to 45°, rotation and sidebending away (FS$_A$R$_A$); C3 is the Maverick point of the cervical spine, meaning it does not follow the typical treatment pattern of the rest of the cervical spine. ✎ Approximately 5% of counterstrain points on the body are Maverick points.	1.1008, 11.39–42

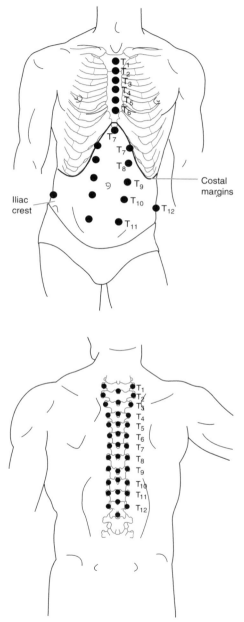

Figure 7–3.

Where are the anterior thoracic tenderpoints for T1-T6 located?

Midline on the sternum at the attachment of the corresponding ribs

1.1009

Where are the anterior tenderpoints for T7-T12 located?

In the rectus abdominus, 1 inch lateral to the midline

1.1009

What is the treatment position for anterior tenderpoints T1-T6?

Flexion of the thorax with internal rotation of the arms

1.1009

True or False: The treatment position for anterior T7-T12 is flexion of the thorax with sidebending and rotation away.

False; T7-T9 is FS_AR_A (flex, sidebend away, rotate away). With T10-T12, the hips are flexed with the legs pulled and rotated to the same side as the tenderpoint.

1.1009–1010

Where are the posterior thoracic tenderpoints located?

Either side of the spinous process or transverse process

1.1009–1010

What is the treatment position for posterior thoracic tenderpoints?

T1-T9: Extension, rotation, and sidebending away

1.1010

T10-T12: Extension of the trunk on the same side as the tenderpoint

Are anterior rib tenderpoints associated with elevated or depressed ribs?

Depressed ribs

1.1011

Which tenderpoints correspond with elevated ribs?

Posterior rib tenderpoints

1.1011

Where are the tenderpoint locations for anterior ribs?

Rib 1: on the first rib at the manubrium

1.1011

Rib 2: on the second rib at the midclavicular line

Rib 3 through 6: on the numbered rib at the anterior axillary line

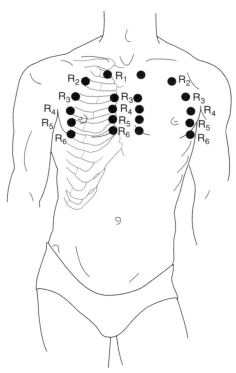

Figure 7–4.

What are the treatment positions for anterior ribs?	Ribs 1 and 2: neck flexion, rotation, and sidebending toward the tenderpoint	1.1011
	Ribs 3 through 6: flexion, elevation of the shoulder, sidebending and rotation toward the tenderpoint	
Where are posterior rib tenderpoints located?	On the posterior aspect of ribs 2 through 6 at the rib angles	1.1012
What is the treatment position for posterior rib tenderpoints?	Flexion, elevation of the shoulder, sidebending, and rotation away from the tenderpoint	1.1012

Counterstrain treatment of ribs is held for what length of time?

120 seconds

1.1011, 11.62–67

Where are the anterior lumbar tenderpoints located?

L1: medial to the anterior superior iliac spine (ASIS)

L2: inferomedial to the AIIS

L3: lateral to the AIIS

L4: inferior to the AIIS

L5: anterior surface of the pubic rami, 1 cm lateral to the symphysis

1.1012

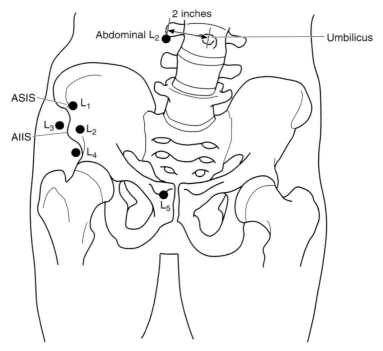

Figure 7–5.

What is the counterstrain treatment position for anterior L1?

Flexion of the hips with knees and feet pulled toward the side of the tenderpoint

1.1012

True or False: The position for treatment of L2-L4 involves standing on the same side as the tenderpoint and flexion of the hips with the knees and feet positioned away from the tenderpoint.

False; the physician stands on the opposite side of the tenderpoint with the knees and feet positioned away from the tenderpoint.

1.1012

What is the counterstrain treatment position for anterior L5?

Flexion of the hips with the knees positioned toward the tenderpoint and feet away from the tenderpoint

1.1012

Where are the posterior L1-L5 tenderpoints located?

On the inferolateral side of the corresponding vertebra's spinous processes

1.1012

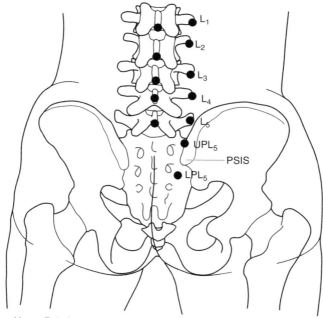

UPL = Upper Pole L$_5$ LPL = Lower Pole L$_5$

Figure 7–6.

What is the counterstrain treatment position for the posterior L1-L5 tenderpoints?	Extension of the trunk on the ipsilateral side of the spinous process	1.1012
Where is the tenderpoint for the iliacus muscle located?	Between the midline and ASIS, 7 cm deep in the abdomen	1.1013
What is the counterstrain treatment position for the iliacus muscle?	Flexion of the hips bilaterally with both hips laterally rotated and knees abducted (frog-leg position)	1.1013
True or False: The lower pole L5 tenderpoint is 2 cm below the posterior superior iliac spine (PSIS).	**True**	1.1013
How is the lower pole L5 tenderpoint treated with counterstrain?	Flexion of the ipsilateral hip to 90° with medial rotation and adduction of the hip	1.1013
Where is the piriformis muscle tenderpoint?	In the piriformis muscle, between the greater trochanter and its attachment to the lateral side of the sacrum	1.1013

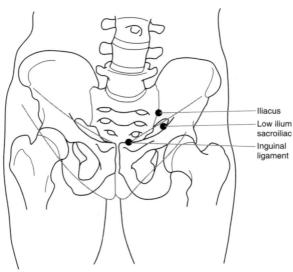

Figure 7–7a.

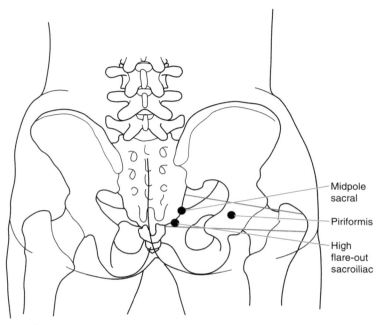

Midpole
sacral

Piriformis

High
flare-out
sacroiliac

☐ Posterior sacral tenderpoints
 overlie the priformis muscle

Figure 7–7b.

What is the piriformis muscle tenderpoint counterstrain treatment position?

Flexion of the ipsilateral hip with   1.1013
abduction and external rotation

Chapter 8

Facilitated Positional Release

What is facilitated positional release (FPR)?	It is an indirect positional treatment method of either abnormal muscle tension or somatic dysfunction.	1.1017
Who developed FPR?	It was developed by Dr. Stanley Schiowitz, D.O.	1.1018
In what position is the patient placed before the physician performs FPR?	The patient is placed in a neutral position, which is a balanced position between flexion and extension.	1.1017
Why is the patient placed in a neutral position for FPR techniques?	To unload the joints' articulating surfaces, allowing the dysfunctional area to respond more easily and rapidly to the applied motion and force	1.1017
Once the patient is in the neutral position, what type of force is applied to perform FPR?	An activating force is applied to encourage immediate release of tissue tension, joint motion restriction, or both.	1.1017
What is the goal of FPR?	To decrease tissue hypertonicity that maintains somatic dysfunction; FPR can also be modified to influence deep muscles involved in joint mobility.	1.1017
What supposedly initiates or maintains the immobility of a dysfunctional segment?	Increased gains in gamma motor neuron activity of the dysfunctional segment	1.1017
How is the patient positioned with FPR?	The anteroposterior (AP) spinal curve of the area that is going to be treated should be flattened.	1.1017–1018

Why is it important to flatten the spine in FPR?	To allow shortening and softening of the involved muscles	1.1017–1018
What is the initial step in FPR?	A facilitating force (compression or torsion) is applied and maintained.	1.1017–1018
Describe the patient's position after the initial step.	The patient's involved myofascial structures are placed in a shortened and relaxed position.	1.1017–1018
Discuss the reasoning behind the positioning of the patient.	This softening of the tissues results in a reduction of stretch receptor activity.	1.1017–1018
How long is the patient held in this position?	This position is held for 3 to 5 seconds and then released; the patient is then re-evaluated.	1.1017–1018
What is the final step in FPR?	The patient's condition is re-evaluated.	1.1017–1018
How would a C5 ES_RR_R diagnosis be treated using FPR?	1. Flatten the cervical lordosis. 2. Place C5 into extension. 3. Sidebend right with respect to C6. 4. Rotate right with respect to C6. 5. Apply the facilitating force. 6. Hold the position for 3 to 5 seconds (*the release should be palpable to the physician*). 7. Re-evaluate the patient.	1.1018
Does it take a long time to perform FPR?	**No;** FPR can be performed in only a few seconds, making it advantageous.	1.1017
In theory, how does FPR immediately affect the muscle spindle-gamma loop?	FPR allows the extrafusal muscle fibers to lengthen to their normal relaxed state compared to the shortened and tense state they experience when somatic dysfunction is present.	1.1017

What is the theoretical reasoning behind shortening a muscle in FPR?

When a muscle is shortened, it causes a decrease in the muscle spindle output and lowers the afferent excitatory input to the spinal cord through the Ia nerve fibers.

1.1017

What is the theoretical result of shortening a muscle in FPR?

With a lowered afferent excitatory input to the spinal cord through the Ia nerve fibers, there is a decrease in gamma motor gain (output) to the spindles and by reflex action, decreased tension of the extrafusal fibers as they lengthen to their more original and normal functioning state.

1.1017

Does all joint motion asymmetry decrease with FPR treatment?

No; only the motions that were impaired by muscle hypertonicity.

1.1017

What are the two main goals of FPR?

1. Normalization of palpable tissue texture
2. Positively influencing the deep muscles involved in joint mobility

1.1018

Chapter 9

Ligamentous Articular Strain

What was the principle demonstrated by A.T. Still on how ligamentous articular release (LAR) strain works?

Exaggeration of the lesion to the degree of release that will allow the ligaments to draw their articulations back into normal relationship

2.13

What are the three basic principles of treating a ligamentous strain with an LAR technique?

1. Disengage, by compression or decompression, until the injured part is able to move.
2. Exaggerate the ligaments back toward the original position of injury until a balance/still point is found.
3. Balance the tension until a release is felt.

Remember **DEB—D**isengage, **E**xaggerate, and **B**alance.

2.25

True or False: In a ligamentous injury, the tighter ligament is usually the injured ligament.

False; the tighter ligament is usually the healthy ligament holding a joint in its place, while the ligament that is more loose is usually the injured ligament.

2.23

Once the joint is returned to its normal physiological position, how long does it take for the ligaments to heal?

About 90 days (3 months), which is the time it takes connective tissue to regenerate; if the joint is not restrained during this period, no further treatment is needed

2.23

Do weakened ligaments allow excess joint motion in the direction of the lesion, or opposite the direction of the lesion?

In the direction of the lesion

2.24

What is indirect LAR?

Carrying the injured body part in the direction that caused the injury

2.25

What is direct LAR?

Carrying the injured body part toward its normal position

2.25

Which technique—direct or indirect—is usually less painful and nontraumatic for the patient?

Indirect LAR techniques

2.26

What is the term for the orientation of ligaments that take on an undulating configuration, allowing the ligaments to work like a spring?

This is known as *crimping*.

2.29

What biochemical changes take place when a ligament is immobilized?

1. Fibrofatty infiltrates increase in the joint capsule.
2. Loss of water and glycosaminoglycans.
3. Optimal distance between fibers decreases.
4. Microadhesions form in a haphazard manner.
5. Joint stiffness increases.

2.29–30

Describe direct myofascial release of the plantar fascia.

It is performed for pain at the bottom of the foot, heel spurs, and plantar fasciitis by contacting the bottom of the foot at the tarsal-metatarsal junction with the thumbs crossed, applying direct pressure toward the sides of the foot and toes.

2.41

Why is the calcaneus technique also described as the "bootjack" technique?

Because the treatment motion is similar to taking a boot off of one's foot

2.44

If a patient's talus is anterior, in which direction should the physician move the tibia when using a direct LAR treatment technique?

The physician should compress the tibia posteriorly into the table with the patient in the supine position; this will move the tibia posteriorly and the talus anteriorly, exaggerating the dysfunction so the involved ligaments once again reset themselves into balance.

2.46

How should a physician treat calf pain and cramping of the foot?

With a supine direct myofascial technique, by pressing the four fingers of each hand side by side into the tight gastrocnemius, compressing the tight muscles, and applying a slight inferior traction

2.49

Describe how to balance the fibular head in a patient with lateral knee pain or an unstable ankle.

Place one hand under the knee, making contact at the fibular head with the thumb and the other hand holding the foot; flex the hip and knee to 90° with slight external rotation of the femur; press the fibular head inferiorly; invert the foot; and balance the tension between the two hands until a release is felt.

2.50

Contacting a posteriorly subluxed meniscus in the popliteal fascia and moving it anteriorly back into its physiologic normal position describes what type of LAR technique?

Moving a posteriorly subluxed meniscus anteriorly into resistance describes a direct LAR technique.

2.55

In which directions should a physician exaggerate a tight iliotibial band in a supine direct myofascial release?

Medial and posterior

2.58

Describe the lateral recumbent direct myofascial release technique of the piriformis.

Very close to its insertion on the femur, slightly posteriorly and inferiorly to the greater trochanter, engage the piriformis muscle and maintain firm pressure with the pads of your thumb medially down into the table.

2.63

Treating the pelvic diaphragm that is stuck downward in exhalation, using a supine direct myofascial release, is indicated with what types of complaints?

Urinary frequency, pain in the rectal area, prostatitis, hemorrhoids, dyspareunia, recurrent urinary tract infections

2.71

Describe how to treat the sacrum with a direct LAR technique.	Have the patient lie in a supine position and reach both hands around to the sacrum, aligning the second- to fifth-digit finger pads along the sacral sulcus; rotate your fingers laterally and your thenar eminences medially.	2.75–76
Where is the iliopsoas muscle located in relation to the femoral artery?	Slightly laterally to the femoral artery	2.80
A spasm in the psoas muscle can be treated by contacting the psoas muscle just laterally to the femoral artery and carrying the muscle which way?	Carrying the iliopsoas muscle laterally will help calm iliopsoas spasms in a direct myofascial release.	2.80
Treating the median umbilical ligament in patients with complaints of urinary frequency involves engaging the ligament halfway between the umbilicus and pubic bone and moving the wrists and hands in what manner?	The physician should rotate the wrists and spread the fingers apart in order to stretch the ligament until a release is felt.	2.85
Treating the umbilicus by rotating it with the pad of one thumb in the direction it prefers is used to treat what complaints?	Abdominal and pelvic pain, gastrointestinal (GI) complaints, and, interestingly, can aid in the treatment of asthma	2.86
Postoperative patients often experience difficulty taking a deep breath. How can a physician treat the thoracoabdominal diaphragm to increase negative intrathoracic pressure and help the patient take a deeper breath?	Place the patient in a supine position engage the abdominal viscera underneath the costal margin, and carry the viscera against the diaphragm until greater diaphragmatic motion and freedom is felt.	2.93

Anterior chest pain is often treated by compressing the sternum and carrying it to a position of ease. Is this an example of a direct or an indirect LAR technique?

Compressing the sternum and carrying it into its ease is an **indirect** LAR technique.

2.94

For lateral chest pain and costochondritis, the patient is placed in a lateral recumbent position and the ribs (4–8) are carried in what direction?

The ribs are carried medially into the table, using a direct LAR technique used more often for bucket handle–motion ribs.

2.96

Describe how to treat ribs 2 through 12 in the supine position.

Disengage the rib anteriorly at the rib angles and then carry them superiorly and laterally; use this technique for chest pain, especially associated with twisting and turning motions.

2.97

What type of myofascial treatment could be used to decrease tension near the terminal portion of the thoracic duct to ensure optimum flow of lymphatic fluid?

A supine direct myofascial release of the anterior cervical fascia; apply a force directly inferiorly into the anterior cervical fascia; when the release is felt, draw the thumbs laterally.

2.113–114

Pain at either end of the clavicle is common in childhood injuries and can be treated by having the patient sit upward, grasping the clavicle at both ends, and moving it in what direction?

Moving the clavicle slightly posteriorly, superiorly, and laterally in a direct LAR technique

2.116

Treating a shoulder that has limited motion involves having the patient laterally recumbent with the injured shoulder up, compressing the shoulder directly in the

Either the anterior *or* the posterior direction

2.118

direction of the opposite glenohumeral joint and balancing the shoulder by moving the shoulder in what direction?

Describe the forearm direct LAR treatment of tennis elbow.

With one hand, flex the wrist and pronate the forearm; with the other hand, grasp the point of the olecrenon between your thumb and index finger; then, compress the forearm between your two hands to the point of balanced tension; and finally draw the elbow into extension, maintaining the other vectors of force.

Hemorrhoids are commonly seen when which diaphragm of the body is not working properly?

The pelvic diaphragm

2.166

What are the eight functional diaphragms of the body (all of which can be treated using LAR or a myofascial release) that must be working together in unison to augment fluid movement throughout the body?

1. Plantar fascia
2. Knee diaphragm (popliteal diaphragm, cruciate ligaments, and transverse ligament of the knee)
3. Pelvic diaphragm
4. Respiratory diaphragm
5. Thoracic outlet (anterior cervical fascia, subclavius muscles, costocoracoid ligaments, and costoclavicular ligaments)
6. Suboccipital triangle
7. Tentorium cerebelli
8. Diaphragm sellae

2.162–163

Chapter 10 — **Muscle Energy**

What is muscle energy?

A form of osteopathic manipulative therapy (OMT) in which patients actively use their own muscles upon the physician's request, *from a precisely controlled position, in a specific direction, against a distinctly executed counterforce* by the physician

1.881

Following a muscle energy treatment, what must one always remember to do?

Recheck the patient's somatic findings to confirm that the dysfunction has been treated and has improved (if not completely resolved)

12.13–15

What is an active treatment?

A treatment during which the patient will **assist** the doctor

12.13–15

What is a direct treatment?

A treatment in which the patient is moved **toward** the barrier

12.13–15

What is an indirect treatment?

A treatment in which the patient is moved **away** from the barrier

12.13–15

Is muscle energy an *active direct* or an *active indirect* technique?

It can be either an active direct or an active indirect technique. For boards, know that most forms of muscle energy are direct techniques.

1.881

What types of patients would not benefit from muscle energy?

1. Comatose patients
2. Uncooperative patients
3. Patients who are too young to cooperate
4. Unresponsive patients

1.881

What are the main treatment goals when using muscle energy?

1. To decrease muscle hypertonicity
2. To lengthen muscle fibers
3. To reduce the restraint of movement

1.881

	4. To produce joint mobilization 5. To improve respiratory and circulatory function 6. To strengthen the weaker side if there is asymmetry	
What physiologic principles are used to accomplish these goals?	1. Postisometric relaxation (direct technique) 2. Reciprocal inhibition (direct and indirect technique) 3. Joint mobilization using muscle force 4. Oculocephalogyric reflex 5. Respiratory assistance 6. Crossed extensor reflex	1.882–883
How is postisometric relaxation theoretically accomplished?	Golgi tendon organs in the muscle tendon sense the change in muscle tension and cause a reflex relaxation of the agonistic muscle fibers; this relaxation allows the physician to passively move the patient toward the new restrictive barrier.	1.882, 6.44
What goals are accomplished when using reciprocal inhibition?	Lengthening of a muscle shortened by a cramp or acute spasm	1.883
What is the physiologic basis behind reciprocal inhibition?	By contracting antagonistic muscles, signals are transmitted to the spinal cord using the reciprocal inhibition reflex arc that force the agonistic muscle to relax.	1.883, 6.45
True or False: Reciprocal inhibition can be done directly or indirectly.	**True;** reciprocal inhibition can be done either directly or indirectly. *Note:* Reciprocal inhibition is also known as reciprocal innervation.	1.883
What is joint mobilization?	Using muscle contractions to establish the joint's normal range of motion	1.882

What is the oculocephalogyric reflex?	A response of the cervical and truncal musculature to voluntary extraocular muscle contractions as the body attempts to follow the lead provided by eye motion	1.882–83
What is a respiratory assistance technique?	A procedure that uses the patient's voluntary respiratory motion to restore normal motion; may involve the direct use of respiratory muscles, or motion transmitted to the spine, pelvis, and extremities	1.88
Will normal respiration be useful if the physician is trying to use a muscle energy technique with respiratory assistance?	Any respiration at all can be useful to a certain degree; however, exaggerated respiration should be suggested for maximal clinical response.	1.883
How does a crossed extensor reflex theoretically work?	Stimulating the agonistic muscle on one side of the body will cause a relaxation of the agonist muscle and contraction of the antagonistic muscle on the opposite side of the body.	1.883, 6.45
What is an example of a crossed extensor reflex?	Flexing the right biceps muscle will cause relaxation of the left biceps and contraction of the left triceps muscle.	6.45
When is a crossed extensor reflex used in muscle energy?	In extremities in which the muscle being treated is so severely injured that it cannot be directly manipulated	1.883
Describe the muscle energy treatment procedure.	1. Engage the restrictive barrier (direct treatment) in all planes of motion. 2. Instruct the patient to move in the reverse direction for one or all planes of motion by	1.884

contracting the appropriate
muscle(s) or muscle group(s).
3. Maintain an appropriate
counterforce.
4. Hold for 3 to 5 seconds.
5. Instruct the patient to relax.
6. Take up the slack.
7. Repeat steps 1 through 6 for
3 to 5 times.

**What must a physician
always do after completing
any technique?**

Recheck the range of motion   1.884

**What takes place when
the physician "takes
up the slack" during the
postisometric relaxation
phase of muscle energy?**

The muscle passively lengthens.   1.884

**What is accomplished by
instructing the patient to
contract appropriate
muscle(s) during muscle
energy?**

Movement of the restricted body   1.884
segment through a complete
range of motion

**When does a satisfactory
response to muscle energy
typically occur?**

About the third time the patient   1.884
is asked to maintain an
appropriate counterforce

**What factors increase the
success of a muscle energy
technique at removing
somatic dysfunction?**

1. Accurate diagnosis   1.884
2. Appropriate levels of force
3. Precise localization

**Is the intensity of force or
localization more important?**

Precise localization of the force   1.884
in **all** planes of motion is more
important than the intensity of
force.

**What critical factor does
precise localization of the
muscle energy force
depend on?**

The physician's palpatory   1.884
perception of movement (or
resistance to movement) at or
about a specific articulation

Why is it important to have good palpatory perception of movement or resistance?

It enables the physician to make subtle assessments about a dysfunction and to create variations of suggested treatment principles.

1.884

True or False: When the physician introduces motion into an articulation that is one or two segments below the dysfunction, the probability of success increases.

False; the probability of success greatly decreases because the forces have not been optimally localized to the restrictive segment.

1.884

What effects can an excessive physician force have on a muscle energy treatment?

Excessive force recruits other muscles to help stabilize the body part being treated and may completely negate the intent of the technique or even cause somatic dysfunction where it was not present before.

1.884

What is the relative contraindication to muscle energy treatments?

Patients with low vitality could be further compromised by adding active muscular exertion.

1.884

Give some examples of patients who cannot be treated with muscle energy.

Postsurgical patients and intensive care patients

1.884

Describe how to treat an occipitoatlantal (OA) ES_LR_R dysfunction with muscle energy.

1. Use the distal pad of one finger and monitor the OA joint.
2. Engage the restrictive barrier in all three planes by sidebending right, rotating left, and flexing the patient's head until tension is felt under the monitoring finger (this is known as localization).
3. Instruct the patient to use a small amount of force to straighten the head.

1.888

4. Simultaneously exert an equal amount of counterforce.
5. Maintain the forces for 3 to 5 seconds.
6. Repeat 3 to 5 times, each time re-engaging the new restrictive barrier.

Describe how to treat an atlantoaxial (AA) R_R dysfunction with muscle energy.

1. Cradle the patient's occiput in your hands.   1.888
2. Flex the patient's cervical spine 45° to lock out all facets below the AA joint.
3. Rotate the atlas to the left until the point of initial resistance is felt.
4. Instruct the patient to gently rotate his/her head to the right.
5. Apply an equal counterforce through your fingers and hands.
6. Maintain the forces for 3 to 5 seconds.
7. Repeat 3 to 5 times, each time re-engaging the new restrictive barrier.

Which joint is treated by using *only* a rotational force?

The AA joint   1.888

Describe how to treat a C3 ER_RS_R dysfunction with muscle energy.

1. Use the distal pad of your finger on the articular pillar of the dysfunctional segment.   1.889
2. Reverse the dysfunction in all three planes of motion until the forces localize under your monitoring finger (rotation and sidebending components are to the same side from C2-C7 in the cervical spine).
3. Instruct the patient to gently straighten her head while you apply an equal counterforce.

4. Maintain the forces for 3 to 5 seconds.
5. Repeat 3 to 5 times, each time re-engaging the new restrictive barrier.

Describe how to treat a T3 ER$_L$S$_L$ dysfunction with muscle energy.

1. In the patient's upper thoracic spine, use his head and neck as a lever to induce motion at the dysfunctional segment.
2. With one hand, monitor the posterior transverse process of T3.
3. Flex, rotate, and sidebend right until the forces are localized under your monitoring finger.
4. Instruct the patient to use a small amount of force to straighten his head while you exert an equal amount of counterforce.
5. Maintain force for 3 to 5 seconds.
6. Ask the patient to relax.
7. Re-engage the new restrictive barrier.
8. Repeat 3 to 5 times, each time re-engaging the new restrictive barrier.

1.886

Describe how to treat a T7 ER$_L$S$_L$ dysfunction with muscle energy.

1. Use your left hand to monitor the posterior transverse process of T7.
2. Instruct the patient to place her left hand behind her neck, and grasp her left elbow with her right hand.
3. Reach across the patient's chest with your right arm.
4. Sidebend and rotate T7 to the right until the forces are localized under your monitoring hand.

1.886

5. Direct the patient to use a small amount of force to straighten her body while you exert an equal amount of counterforce.
6. Repeat 3 to 5 times, each time re-engaging the new restrictive barrier.

What are the restricted motions of a T4 ER$_L$S$_L$ dysfunction?

There is restriction of flexion, right rotation, and right sidebending at T4.

1.886

If a patient has restriction in left rotation and right sidebending at segments T5-T9, how would these findings be recorded?

T5-T9 NR$_R$S$_L$

1.886

What is a key rib?

The major restrictor of the rib group's ability to move into inhalation or exhalation. This rib always leads to dysfunctional movement, dragging successive ribs behind.

1.723

What is a rib dysfunction (rib lesion)?

A type of somatic dysfunction in which movement or position of one or several ribs is altered or disrupted

1.1245

What is the key rib in an exhalation rib dysfunction?

The ribs are held downward; therefore the key rib is the top rib of the dysfunctional group and should be the first rib treated.

1.1245

What is the key rib in an inhalation rib dysfunction?

The ribs are held upward; therefore the key rib is the bottom rib of the dysfunctional group and should be the first rib treated.

1.1245

Which rib should be treated first if a group of ribs is found to be held in exhalation?

The key rib is the top rib of the dysfunctional group and should be the first rib treated.

1.890

Why is this rib treated first?

Because the top rib of the dysfunctional group may also be pushing several of the ribs below it downward

1.890

Describe the rib motion of a first rib inhalation dysfunction.

The first rib elevates fully with inhalation but does not move much with exhalation.

1.891

In what position is the patient placed when performing muscle energy to correct an elevated right first rib dysfunction?

Seated on the side of the table with the left arm draped over the physician's thigh

1.891

Where should the physician stand when using muscle energy to correct an elevated right first rib?

Behind the patient; the physician's left foot should be on the table next to the patient's hip.

1.891

Describe how to treat an elevated right first rib dysfunction with muscle energy.

1. The metacarpophalangeal (MCP) joint of the physician's right index finger contacts the upper surface of the dysfunctional rib, posteriorly and laterally to the costotransverse articulation.
2. The physician's left hand guides the patient's head forward, sidebends and rotates the patient's head away from the side of the dysfunction.
3. The physician instructs the patient to inhale and exhale deeply.
4. As the patient exhales, the physician exerts a caudal and forward pressure on the superior surface of the rib, resisting the inhalation motion of the first rib.
5. The physician then instructs the patient to take 3 to 7 cycles of respiration.

1.891

When treating an elevated right first rib with muscle energy, the physician will guide the patient's head forward, sidebend and rotate it away from the dysfunction. What is the purpose of these motions?

To take tension off the scalene muscles

1.890

When does a physician know that an elevated right first rib has been improved with muscle energy?

When maximal motion of the dysfunctional rib has been obtained

1.890

In what position is the patient placed when performing muscle energy to correct an inhalation dysfunction of rib 4?

The supine position

1.890

Describe how to treat an inhalation dysfunction of ribs 2 through 6 with muscle energy.

1. Place one hand on the anterior aspect of the lower key rib.
2. Flex the patient for pump handle dysfunctions (sidebend the patient for bucket handle dysfunctions) down to the dysfunctional rib to remove the tension.
3. Instruct the patient to inhale and then exhale deeply.
4. Instruct the patient to hold his breath at the end of the expiratory phase for 3 to 5 seconds.
5. During this time, adjust flexion/sidebending to the new restrictive barrier.
6. Follow the rib shaft into exhalation with your hand during the expiratory phase.
7. On inhalation, the physician resists the inhalation motion of the rib.
8. Repeat 3 to 5 times.

1.890

When treating bucket handle dysfunctions, what is the patient instructed to do before holding her breath in expiration for 3 to 5 seconds?	The patient is instructed to reach for her knee on the affected side.	1.891
Which muscles are used to treat an exhalation dysfunction of rib 1?	The anterior and middle scalene muscles	3.565
Which muscle is used to treat an exhalation dysfunction of rib 2?	The posterior scalene muscle	3.565
Which muscle is used to treat an exhalation dysfunction of ribs 3-5?	The pectoralis minor muscle	3.565
Which muscle is used to treat an exhalation dysfunction of ribs 6-9?	The serratus anterior muscle	3.565
Which muscle is used to treat an exhalation dysfunction of ribs 10 and 11?	The latissimus dorsi muscle *Note:* Ribs 11 and 12 can be treated with the quadratus lumborum.	3.565
Which muscle is used to treat an exhalation dysfunction of rib 12?	The quadratus lumborum muscle	3.565
Describe how to treat exhalation rib dysfunctions with muscle energy.	1. The patient is instructed to place his forearm on the dysfunctional side across his forehead with his palm facing up. 2. Grasp the key rib posteriorly at the rib angle. 3. Instruct the patient to inhale deeply while applying an inferior traction on the rib angle.	1.892–1.893

4. Instruct patient to hold his breath at full inhalation while performing one of the following isometric contractions for 3 to 5 seconds:

Rib 1: Patient raises his head directly toward the ceiling.

Rib 2: Patient turns his head 30° away from the dysfunctional side and lifts his head toward the ceiling.

Ribs 3 through 5: Patient pushes his elbow on the dysfunctional side toward the opposite anterior superior iliac spine (ASIS).

Ribs 6 through 9: Patient pushes his arm anteriorly.

Ribs 10 through 12: Patient adducts his arm.

5. Repeat 3 to 5 times, each time re-engaging the new restrictive barrier.

How is the patient positioned for muscle energy of the lumbar spine?

The patient is placed in the seated position.

1.885

Describe how to treat an L3 ES$_R$R$_R$ dysfunction with muscle energy.

In the same manner as the lower thoracic spine

1.885

What information is required for diagnosing sacral dysfunction?

Two types of information are needed:
The position of the two sacral sulci and the two inferior lateral angles (ILA), in addition to the results of (this test is a procedure by which information is obtained) a motion test

1.897

	The results of a seated and/or standing flexion test	
What tests can be used to screen for a unilateral sacroiliac dysfunction?	1. Lumbar spring test 2. Sphinx test 3. Seated flexion test 4. Seated assessment of ILA asymmetry	1.897
In what position is the patient placed when performing muscle energy to correct a right unilateral sacral extension?	The patient is placed in the prone position.	1.897
Describe how to treat a unilateral sacral dysfunction with muscle energy.	1. Place your left hypothenar eminence on the patient's right sacral sulcus. 2. Ask the patient to exhale and hold her breath while you push anteriorly and caudad on her superior sulcus. 3. Hold for 3 to 5 seconds. 4. Direct the patient to inhale while you resist any anterior superior movement of the sacrum. 5. Repeat 3 to 5 times.	1.899–1.900
Is a L on L sacral dysfunction considered a backward or forward torsion?	**Forward** sacral torsion	1.898
To what position is the patient rotated when performing muscle energy to correct a L on L sacral torsion?	Forward sacral torsion → The patient is rotated so that her/his chest faces down (**forward** onto the treatment table)	1.898
Describe how to treat a L on L sacral dysfunction with muscle energy.	1. The patient lies on his left side (axis side down) with his torso rotated so the patient's face is down. 2. Flex the patient's hips until the motion localizes at the lumbosacral junction.	1.898–1.899

3. Drop the patient's legs off table to induce left sidebending and engage a left sacral oblique axis.
4. Ask the patient to lift his legs toward ceiling against an equal counterforce for 3 to 5 seconds.
5. Monitor the right superior pole of the sacrum for posterior movement with your other hand.
6. Repeat for 3 to 5 times.

What type of torsion is a R on L sacral dysfunction?

Backward sacral torsion

1.899

In what position is the patient rotated when performing muscle energy for a R on L sacral torsion?

The patient is lying on her left side (axis side down) with torso rotated so that she is facing upward with her back on the treatment table.

1.899

Note: When patients are being treated for a **back**ward (non-neutral) torsion, they are placed on their **backs.**

Describe how to treat a R on L sacral torsion with muscle energy.

1. Grasp the patient's left arm and pull inferiorly to rotate his torso to the right.
2. Flex the patient's hips until motion is localized at the lumbosacral junction.
3. Drop the patient's legs off the table to induce left sidebending and engage a left sacral oblique axis.
4. Ask the patient to lift his legs toward the ceiling against an equal counterforce for 3 to 5 seconds.
5. Monitor the right superior pole for anterior movement with your other hand.

1.899

6. Repeat for 3 to 5 times, each time re-engaging the new restrictive barrier.

What causes innominate dysfunction?

Irregularities in the biomechanics of the sacroiliac joint

1.894

What maintains innominate somatic dysfunction?

Ligamentous tension

1.894

What is the role of muscle energy in innominate dysfunction?

To restore normal articular relations across the sacroiliac joint

1.895

Describe how to treat a right anterior innominate dysfunction with muscle energy.

1. Flex the patient's right hip and knee until resistance is felt.
2. Instruct the patient to extend his/her hip against a counter-force for 3 to 5 seconds.
3. Wait a few seconds for the tissues to relax.
4. Take up the slack to the new restrictive barrier.
5. Repeat until no restrictive barrier is felt (3 to 5 times).

1.895

If an innominate is rotated anterior, what is the restriction?

Posterior innominate rotation

1.895

How is a right innominate anterior treated differently than a right innominate posterior?

Right innominate anterior:
Patient flexes right hip and knee.

Patient extends hip against a counterforce.

Right innominate posterior:
Patient's right leg is dropped off the table and abducts.

Patient flexes and adducts knee against counterforce.

1.895

When treating a right anterior innominate dysfunction, is the patient supine or prone?	The patient is placed in the **supine** position.	1.895
When treating a right posterior innominate dysfunction, is the patient supine or prone?	The patient is placed in the supine position.	1.895
What type of patient history would lead a physician suspect an abducted pubic bone?	Recent childbirth or surgery performed in the lithotomy position *Note:* The lithotomy position is the position where a women is placed on her back with her knees bent and thighs apart; it is assumed for vaginal or rectal examination, and sometimes for childbearing.	1.896
How do patients with abducted pubic bones usually present?	Because of fascia stresses placed on the urethra, some patients experience urinary frequency and urgency suggestive of infectious cystitis. *Note:* Laboratory studies do not support this diagnosis.	1.895
In what position is the patient placed when performing muscle energy to correct abducted pubic bones?	The patient is placed supinely with hips flexed to 45°, knees flexed to 90°, and feet flat on the table.	1.897
Describe how to treat abducted pubic bones with muscle energy.	1. The patient's knees are separated about 18 inches. 2. The lateral aspect of the knee closest to the physician is placed against the physician's abdomen (using a pillow to protect the physician). 3. Reach across the other knee and grasp the lateral aspect of that knee with both hands.	1.897

4. The patient is then asked to pull his knees apart as hard as he can against the physician's counterforce.
5. Hold for 3 to 5 seconds.
6. Ask the patient to relax and wait 2 seconds for the tissues to relax.
7. Pull the knees slightly closer together.
8. Repeat 3 to 5 times.

What are the differences between treating a right superior pubic shear and treating a right inferior pubic shear with muscle energy?

Right superior pubic shear: 1.897
   1. The patient's right leg is off the table and abducted.
   2. The patient is instructed to bring the right knee to his/her left ASIS.

Right inferior pubic shear:
   1. The patient's right hip and knee are flexed and abducted.
   2. The patient is instructed to extend and adduct the right knee.

Describe how to treat a posterior radial head dysfunction with muscle energy.

1. The physician places his right   1.897
   hand at the distal end of the patient's right forearm.
2. Supinate the forearm to resistance while monitoring with your other thumb at the radial head.
3. Instruct the patient to pronate his/her forearm to the right against an equal counterforce supplied by physician's right hand.
4. Hold for 3 to 5 seconds.
5. Relax.
6. Take up the slack to a new point of resistance.
7. Repeat for 3 to 5 times.

How is motion of the forearm affected when the patient has a right posterior radial head?

The patient's right forearm has   1.900
restriction with supination.

Chapter 11

The High Velocity, Low Amplitude Technique

Is the high velocity, low amplitude (HVLA) technique an active or a passive technique?	HVLA is a **passive** treatment technique.	1.852
Is HVLA a direct or an indirect technique?	HVLA is a **direct** treatment technique.	1.852
What are thrust techniques?	A collection of direct manipulative treatments that use HVLA activation	1.852
What is another name for HVLA (that may sound less abrasive)?	Mobilization with impulse	1.852
What is the goal of HVLA?	To move a dysfunctional segment through its restrictive barrier so that the joint **resets itself**	1.852
What is accomplished when a joint resets itself after treatment with HVLA?	Restoration of physiologic motion	1.852
When is the thrust administered in HVLA?	After precise positioning of the dysfunctional segment against the restrictive barrier	1.852
How is an HVLA thrust best described?	A short (low-amplitude), quickly (high-velocity) executed force	1.852
What sign is most commonly associated with an effective thrust technique?	Ordinarily, a click or pop is heard at the time the force is applied.	1.852

True or False: The pop or click after an HVLA thrust indicates that the restricted joint is now "fixed."

False; although a noise is usually indicative of success, it is possible that an unrelated joint may have made the noise and the restricted joint remained unaltered.

1.855

Note: Always retest motion after treatment.

What is the normal physiologic reaction to a painful hypermobile joint?

Muscles surrounding the joint protect it from excess motion by splinting the joint; a physical examination would reveal restriction of motion at the dysfunctional segment.

1.854

True or False: HVLA can be used every time there is an unstable hypermobile joint.

False; although HVLA may work as evidenced by a decrease in pain and improvement in motion, the more it is used, the looser the joint becomes, possibly leading eventually to an unstable joint.

1.854

Describe the proper management of an unstable hypermobile joint.

1. Modify the activity that contributes to the instability.
2. Mobilize less mobile adjacent joints.
3. Prescribe active rehabilitation exercises.

1.854

What maintains the restricted joint motion at a dysfunctional segment?

Abnormal muscle activity known as hypertonicity

1.855

What are the indications for HVLA?

1. Restriction of joint motion
2. Conclusion by the physician that treatment of the joint restriction will benefit the patient

1.855

When are thrust techniques not indicated for treating lost motion seen with somatic dysfunction?

When a restricted segment is the result of an abnormal anatomic or pathologic change, such as a traumatic contracture, advanced

1.855

degenerative joint disease, or ankylosis

Note: Think of the risk/benefit relationship.

True or False: Thrust techniques are most effective and should be used when the barrier feels rubbery and indistinct.

False; the barrier must feel solid, with an abrupt and discernible end point.

1.855

When using a thrust technique, what happens to the excess force not used in moving the dysfunctional joint past its restrictive barrier?

It is dissipated to other parts of the body, which can result in iatrogenic side effects.

1.855

Note: The patient will experience the least iatrogenic side effects if the physician is most specific and accurate at localizing the impulse force vectors, in addition to using the minimal force necessary in taking the joint past its restrictive barrier.

True or False: Once the barrier is engaged, the thrust should be applied without backing off of the restriction.

True; do not back off before delivering the corrective thrust and do not carry the force through a great distance.

1.856

True or False: Amplitude (in reference to osteopathic treatment techniques) refers to the amount of applied force.

False; amplitude refers to the treatment distance of the applied force.

1.856

How can a physician improve the effectiveness of an HVLA technique?

By instructing the patient to relax and diverting his/her attention just before applying the corrective force

1.856

What problems can occur from performing HVLA on a tense patient?

A greater force would be needed to overcome the barrier, thus increasing the chance for side effects and an unsuccessful treatment.

1.856

What are signs that HVLA might be hurting the patient?	Nonverbal cues, such as a facial grimace and the presence of involuntary muscle tightening, known as guarding	1.856
True or False: Older and younger patients usually respond similarly to HVLA.	**False;** older patients respond more slowly to HVLA, while response to HVLA in younger patients is relatively quicker.	1.856
During what phase of respiration should the physician administer the HVLA thrust?	During the exhalation phase of respiration	1.856
True or False: Daily use of HVLA on a patient is good osteopathic practice that will ensure the treated somatic dysfunction does not reoccur.	**False;** a physician needs to be compassionate and give the patient time to respond to the treatment. Sicker patients usually need more time between treatments. *Note:* Daily treatment is excessive for any patient.	1.856
What major complications may occur when using thrust techniques?	1. Permanent neurologic damage 2. Vertebral basilar thrombosis 3. Death (or quadriplegia) from rupturing/weakening of the transverse ligament of the atlas	1.856
What guidelines can be followed to ensure patient safety when using HVLA?	1. Be aware of possible complications. 2. Make an accurate diagnosis. 3. Palpatory examination is a prerequisite. 4. Listen with hands and fingers (if it does not feel right, collect more data). 5. Emphasize specificity. 6. Ask for permission to treat. 7. If the patient is not responding to treatment, re-evaluate. 8. Be aware of the total picture.	1.857

In what position should the patient be placed when treating an occipitoatlantal (OA) FS_RR_L dysfunction?

The patient is placed in the supine position. 1.857

Where should the physician be located when treating an OA FS_RR_L dysfunction?

At the head of the table 1.857

Describe how to treat an OA FS_RR_L dysfunction with HVLA.

1. Grasp the patient's head. 1.857
2. Flex the neck slightly.
3. The physician's metacarpalphalangeal (MCP) joint of the thrusting hand is placed at the base of the patient's occiput.
4. Slightly extend the occiput, limiting the extension to the OA joint.
5. Sidebend the occiput to the left and rotate to the right.

Describe the direction of the HVLA thrust used when treating an OA FS_RR_L dysfunction.

Translate the occiput to the right and direct the HVLA thrust towards the patient's opposite (right) eye. 1.857

What must the physician always do after completing any osteopathic procedure?

Re-evaluate the range of motion 1.857

If a patient's atlas is rotated to the right in relationship to the axis, how is this recorded by an osteopathic physician?

AA R_R 1.857

In what position should the patient be placed when treating an AA R_R dysfunction?

The patient is placed in the supine position. 1.857

Where should the physician be when located treating an AA R_R dysfunction?

At the head of the table 1.857

Describe how to treat an AA R$_R$ dysfunction with HVLA.	1. The physician grasps the patient's chin with the physician's left palm. 2. The physician's right index finger is placed by the AA joint. 3. The physician's thumb contacts the patient's zygomatic process.	1.857
Describe the direction of the HVLA thrust used when treating an AA R$_R$ dysfunction.	It is applied in a left rotational pattern, using the right index finger as a fulcrum.	1.857
In what phase of respiration is the HVLA thrust applied?	At the end of exhalation	1.857
Describe the type of HVLA thrusts used when treating the cervical spine (C2-C7).	Sidebending or rotational thrusts	1.858
In what position is the patient placed when performing HVLA to correct a C3 FS$_L$R$_L$ dysfunction?	The patient is placed in the supine position.	1.858
Where does the physician stand when performing rotational HVLA to treat a C3 FS$_L$R$_L$ dysfunction?	To the right side of the patient, at the head of the table	1.858
Describe how to treat a C3 FS$_L$R$_L$ dysfunction with HVLA.	1. Grasp the patient's head. 2. Slightly flex the neck. 3. Place the MCP joint of the thrusting hand at the articular pillar of C3. 4. Flex both the head and neck to C3. 5. Slightly extend the neck by applying an anterior translation at C3. 6. Rotate the head and neck to the restrictive barrier. 7. Sidebend the head and neck to the right.	1.858

Describe the direction of the HVLA thrust used when treating a C3 FS_LR_L dysfunction.

Using the left MCP joint as a fulcrum, the thrust is applied toward the patient's opposite eye.

1.858

In what position is the patient placed when performing HVLA for a C6 ES_RR_R dysfunction?

The patient is placed in the supine position.

1.858–859

Describe how to treat a C6 ES_RR_R dysfunction with HVLA.

1. The left MCP joint is placed at the articular pillar of C6.
2. Flex the head and neck to the C6-C7 joint.
3. Add a small amount of extension by applying an anterior translation at C6.
4. Sidebend the neck left.
5. Localize at the C6-C7 joint.
6. Rotate neck to the right to lock the above facets.

1.858–859

Describe the direction of the HVLA thrust used when treating a C6 ES_RR_R dysfunction.

Translate C6 to the R to sidebend the HVLA thrust. Direct the activating force toward the patient's opposite shoulder.

1.858–859

True or False: The thoracic spine and ribs can effectively be treated with HVLA only when the patient is placed in the supine position.

False; the thoracic spinal segments and ribs can be treated using HVLA with the patient positioned in multiple positions.

1.859

Where is the corrective thrust directed when treating an extended thoracic lesion?

At the thoracic spinal vertebrae below the dysfunctional segment, with the thrust aimed 45° cephalad and posterior at the fulcrum

1.860

How do you treat a neutral thoracic lesion using HVLA?

In the same manner as a flexed dysfunction; however, the patient is sidebent *away* from the physician.

1.860

When using HVLA on a purely flexed thoracic spinal cord lesion, in what direction should the patient be sidebent?	Away from the physician	1.860
When using HVLA on a purely extended thoracic spinal lesion, in what direction should the patient be sidebent?	Away from the physician	1.860
When using HVLA, describe the placement of the physician's hand and the setup of a purely flexed or extended thoracic spinal cord lesion?	1. Make a bilateral fulcrum using the thenar eminence and flexing the fingers of your caudal hand. 2. Straddle the spinous processes. 3. Contact the soft paraspinal tissues over both transverse processes at the level of the dysfunctional segment.	1.860
Describe the direction of the HVLA thrust used when treating a flexed thoracic lesion.	Towards the floor (posterior) at the level of the dysfunctional thoracic spinal segment	1.860–861
In what position is the patient placed when performing HVLA for an $S_R R_R$ diagnosis?	The patient is placed in the supine position.	1.860–861
Where should the physician stand when using HVLA to treat a T7 $FS_R R_R$ dysfunction?	On the left side of the patient (the opposite side of the posterior transverse process)	1.860–861
Describe the procedure for using HVLA to treat a T7 $FS_R R_R$ dysfunction after the patient has properly been set up for the technique.	1. Cross the patient's arms over his chest (superior arm should be opposite that of the physician; "opposite *over* adjacent"). 2. The physician's thenar eminence (fulcrum) is placed under the posterior transverse process of the dysfunctional segment.	1.860–861

3. The physician's other hand flexes the patient's torso to the T7-T8 joint space.
4. Sidebend the patient to the left, engaging the restrictive barrier.

Describe the HVLA thrust used to treat a T7 FS_RR_R dysfunction.

Straight down (posterior) through the thenar eminence, toward the floor

1.860–861

What does a diagnosis of T5 FS_RR_R indicate?

It indicates that T5 easily sidebends to the right and rotates to the right in relationship to T6; this can also be stated as T5 is restricted in both sidebending and rotation to the left in relationship to T6.

1.860

In what position is the patient placed when performing HVLA to correct a T7 NS_LR_R dysfunction?

The patient is placed in the supine position.

1.860

Where should the physician stand when using HVLA to treat a T7 NS_LR_R dysfunction?

On the left side of the patient (opposite the posterior transverse process)

1.860

Describe how to treat a T7 NS_LR_R dysfunction with HVLA.

1. Cross the patient's arms opposite over adjacent.
2. The physician's thenar eminence is placed under the posterior transverse process of the dysfunctional segment.
3. The physician's other hand is used to flex the patient's torso to the T7-T8 joint space.
4. Sidebend the patient to the right (away from physician) to engage the restrictive barrier.

1.860

Describe the direction of the HVLA thrust used when treating a T7 NS_LR_R dysfunction.	Straight down (posterior) through the thenar eminence, towards the floor, produced more by a momentary drop of one's body weight than by compression of the patient	1.860–861
What are the absolute contraindications for using HVLA?	1. Osteoporosis 2. Osteomyelitis 3. Fractures in the area of thrust 4. Bone metastasis 5. Severe rheumatoid arthritis 6. Down syndrome	1.852–855
Where should the physician stand when using HVLA to treat a first rib inhalation dysfunction with the patient in the supine position?	At the head of the table if placing the patient in the supine position	1.864
Describe how to set up and properly position a patient for HVLA treatment of a first rib inhalation dysfunction with the patient in the supine position.	1. The physician's first MCP is placed on the tubercle of the first rib. 2. Rotate the head and neck away from the side of the dysfunctional rib. 3. Sidebend the head and neck to the side of the dysfunctional rib.	1.864
Describe the direction of the HVLA thrust used when treating a first rib inhalation dysfunction with the patient supine.	1. The thrust is through the thenar eminence. 2. The directions are medial, inferior, and posterior.	1.864
What does the diagnosis of a first rib inhalation dysfunction mean?	The first rib is held cephalad upon expiration instead of correctly moving caudad.	1.864
In what positions can a patient be placed to perform HVLA on a first rib dysfunction?	The supine, seated, and prone positions may all be used.	1.865

In what position is the patient placed when performing HVLA to correct a right rib 5 inhalation dysfunction?

The patient can be placed in either the supine or prone positions; we will discuss the supine positioning below.

1.866–867

In what position is the patient placed when performing HVLA to correct a right rib 5 exhalation dysfunction?

The patient can be placed in either the supine or prone positions; we will discuss the supine positioning below.

1.866–867

Where should the physician stand when using HVLA to treat a right rib 5 inhalation or exhalation dysfunction?

On the left side of the patient (the opposite side from the dysfunctional rib)

1.866–867

True or False: A right rib 5 inhalation dysfunction is treated in a similar manner to a right rib 5 exhalation dysfunction.

True; both rib dysfunctions are treated in a similar manner.

1.866–867

Describe how to treat a right rib 5 inhalation or exhalation dysfunction using HVLA with the patient in the supine position.

1. Stand on the opposite side from the dysfunctional rib.
2. Cross the patient's arms **opposite over adjacent.**
3. The thenar eminence of the physician's cephalic hand is placed under the posterior rib angle of the key rib.
4. The physician's caudal hand is used to flex the patient's torso and sidebend the patient away from the dysfunctional rib.

1.866–867

Describe the direction of the HVLA thrust used when treating a right rib 5 inhalation dysfunction.

Straight down (posterior) through the thenar eminence, toward the floor

1.866–867

What is the rib's motion in an exhalation rib dysfunction?

The dysfunctional rib is held downward; it moves freely down during expiration but fails to move upward (is restricted) during inhalation.

1.866

What is the rib's motion in an inhalation rib dysfunction?

The dysfunctional rib is held upward; it moves freely upward during inhalation but fails to move downward (is restricted) during exhalation.

1.866

What is a key rib?

A key rib is the rib to which treatment should be directed when a group dysfunction of the ribs is present because it is the rib thought to be causing the rest of the ribs to be dysfunctional.

1.866

With what technique are spinal levels T10-L5 traditionally treated when using HVLA?

It is a treatment technique commonly referred to as the "lumbar roll."

1.869

True or False: When treating flexion, extension, and neutral lesions of spinal levels T10-L5 with the lumbar roll technique, patients are always placed in the same position.

True; flexion, extension, and neutral lesions of spinal levels T10-L5 can all be treated with the patient placed in a lateral recumbent position.

1.869

When using the lumbar roll technique to treat flexion/ extension and neutral lesions of spinal levels T10-L5, should the physician place the patient so that the posterior transverse process is directed up or directed down?

The physician may treat the patient with the posterior transverse process up or down.

1.868–870

With respect to the direction the patient's inferior arm is pulled, what is the only difference between the two HVLA treatments (treating the patient with his/her posterior transverse process up and treating the patient with his\her posterior transverse process down)?

Type I (neutral) dysfunction:
Transverse process up = pull the patient's inferior arm up

Transverse process down = pull the patient's inferior arm down

1.869–870

Type II (non-neutral) dysfunction:

Transverse process up = pull the patient's inferior arm down

Transverse process down = pull the patient's inferior arm up

In what position is the patient placed when performing HVLA on a L on L sacral dysfunction?

The patient is placed in the left lateral recumbent position.

1.870

Where should the physician stand when using HVLA to treat a L on L sacral dysfunction?

The physician stands facing the patient.

1.871

In what position is the patient placed when performing HVLA on an anterior rotated innominate?

The patient is placed in the lateral recumbent position.

1.871

Where should the physician stand when using HVLA to treat an anterior rotated innominate?

The physician stands facing the patient.

1.872

Describe how to treat an anterior rotated innominate dysfunction with HVLA.

1. Flex the patient's legs to 90°.
2. Drop the patient's upper leg over the lower leg, making sure the patient's upper leg is also off the table.
3. Contact the ilium with the physician's caudal forearm between the posterior superior iliac spine (PSIS) and the greater trochanter.
4. The thenar eminence of the physician's cephalic hand is placed on the patient's anterior superior iliac spine (ASIS).
5. Use the cephalic hand to carry the patient's shoulder backward until localization has occurred against the restrictive barrier.

1.873

Describe the direction of the HVLA thrust used when treating an anterior rotated innominate.

A rotary thrust down the shaft of the femur; because the thrust is below the axis of rotation, the innominate rotates posterior.

1.873

In what position is the patient placed when performing HVLA on an upslipped innominate (superior iliac shear)?

The patient is placed in the supine position.

1.874

Where should the physician stand when using HVLA to treat an upslipped innominate?

The physician stands at the patient's feet.

1.874

Describe how to treat an upslipped innominate dysfunction with HVLA.

1. Grasp the patient's leg on the dysfunctional side, superior to the ankle.
2. Flex the patient's leg.
3. Apply traction and internally rotate the leg.

1.874

Describe the direction of the HVLA thrust used when treating an upslipped innominate.

1. Ask the patient to relax the affected knee and hip.
2. Use tractional force to the leg.

1.874

Where should the physician stand when using HVLA to treat a posterior radial head?

The physician is on the dysfunctional side of the patient.

1.874

Describe how to treat a posterior radial head dysfunction with HVLA.

1. The physician's thumb is placed over the posterolateral aspect of the patient's radial head.
2. Grasp the patient's wrist with your other hand (thumb is over the dorsum of the patient's distal ulna).
3. Supinate the patient's wrist and extend the patient's elbow at the same time.

1.874

Describe the direction of the HVLA thrust used when treating a posterior radial head.

Apply force on the radial head through the physician's thumb, in a ventral direction.

1.874

How does a patient with a posterior radial head dysfunction usually present?

1. There is tenderness over the radial head.
2. The radial head moves freely with pronation.
3. The radial head is posterior.
4. The radial head is restricted in anterior glide.

1.874

What is the goal of treating an anterior fibular head?

To increase the posterior glide of the restricted fibular head

1.876

Describe how to treat an anterior fibular head dysfunction with HVLA.

1. Place a pillow below the patient's dysfunctional knee to avoid locking it in extension.
2. Grasp the patient's leg immediately proximally to the ankle with the physician's caudal hand.
3. The thenar eminence of the physician's cephalic hand is placed on the anterior aspect of the patient's fibular head.
4. Internally rotate the patient's ankle to draw the distal fibula anterior.

1.876

Describe the direction of the HVLA thrust used when treating an anterior fibular head.

1. Using the cephalic hand, apply a posterolateral force to the fibular head.
2. Simultaneously apply a slight internal rotational counterforce to the ankle using the caudal hand.

1.876

Chapter 12

Cranial Techniques and Osteopathy in the Cranial Field

What are the five components of the primary respiratory mechanism (PRM)?

1. Inherent mobility of the brain and spinal cord
2. Fluctuation of the cerebrospinal fluid (CSF)
3. Movement of the intraspinal and intracranial membranes
4. Articular mobility of the cranial bones
5. Involuntary mobility of the sacrum between the ilia

1.986–989, 10.177–178

How is the inherent motion of the brain and spinal cord described?

A subtle, slow pulse–wave-like movement

1.986–987

What happens to the brain and spinal cord during the exhalation phase?

They lengthen and thin.

1.986–987

What are the three intracranial and intraspinal membranes that surround, support, and protect the CNS?

1. The dura mater
2. The arachnoid mater
3. The pia mater

1.987

Where are the firm attachments of the dura mater located as it descends down the spinal cord?

Around the foramen magnum, C2, C3, and S2

1.987–990

The rocking motion of the sacrum in response to the movement of the dural membrane occurs about which axis?

Superior transverse axis, also known as the respiratory axis

1.987–990

During which phase of respiration do the brain and spinal cord shorten and thicken?	The inhalation phase	1.986–987
In what way do the midline bones move in response to the pull of the dural membrane?	Flexion and extension	1.987–990
Which bones move through an external/internal rotation phase in response to the pull of the dural membrane?	The paired bones of the cranium	1.987–990
What is the significance of the sphenobasilar synchondrosis (SBS)?	The SBS is the articulation of the sphenoid with the occiput in response to the pull of the dural membrane.	1.987–990
Which bones are known as the unpaired midline bones?	The sphenoid, occiput, ethmoid, and vomer	1.987–990
When the SBS flexes, what cardinal movement of the midline and paired bones occurs?	The midline bones also flex as the paired bones move into external rotation.	1.990–991
What happens to the anteroposterior (AP) diameter of the heads when the midline bones are flexed?	The AP diameter of the head decreases with flexion of the midline bones; the transverse diameter of the head increases (widens).	1.990–991
When the SBS flexes, does the sacral base move posterior or anterior?	With flexion of the SBS, the sacral base moves posterior as the dura is pulled cephalad.	1.990–991
When the midline bones extend, what motion takes place with the paired bones?	The paired bones will move into internal rotation, and the head will increase in AP diameter and decrease in transverse diameter.	1.990–991

When the SBS extends, does the sacral base move posterior or anterior?

With extension of the SBS, the sacral base moves anterior as the dura drops in a caudal direction.

1.990–991

Describe what happens functionally (to the midline bones, the sacral base, the AP diameter of the head, motion of the paired bones, brain and spinal cord dimensions, and the slope of the forehead) during craniosacral flexion.

1. Flexion at the SBS as well as the midline bones
2. Posterior movement of the sacral base, also known as counternutation
3. Decreased AP diameter of the head
4. External rotation of the paired bones
5. Shortening and thickening of the brain and spinal cord
6. Increase in the slope of the forehead

1.987–991

Describe what happens functionally (to the midline bones, the sacral base, the AP diameter of the head, motion of the paired bones, brain and spinal cord dimensions, and the slope of the forehead) during craniosacral extension.

1. Extension at the SBS as well as the midline bones
2. Anterior movement of the sacral base, also known as nutation
3. Increased AP diameter of the head
4. Internal rotation of the paired bones
5. Lengthening and thickening of the brain and spinal cord
6. Decrease in the slope of the forehead, creating the appearance of frontal bossing

1.987–991

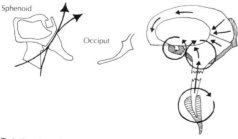

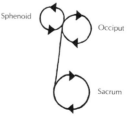

Relationship of sphenoid to occiput

Effects on reciprocal tension membrane system

Direction of force in flexion

Figure 12–1.

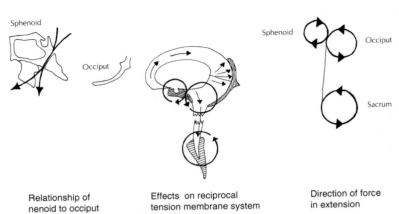

Relationship of
nenoid to occiput

Effects on reciprocal
tension membrane system

Direction of force
in extension

Figure 12–2.

What is the cranial rhythmic impulse (CRI)?	It is the palpatory sensation of the skull widening and narrowing; this sensation is the result of the five components of the PRM.	10.177
What is the rate of the CRI?	Although this is a widely debated question, **for boards** know that the rate of the CRI is 8 to 14 times per minute.	1.991, 10.177
What factors may increase the rate and quality of the CRI?	1. Vigorous physical exercise 2. Systemic effects 3. Effective osteopathic manipulative therapy (OMT) of the craniosacral mechanism	1.991, 10.177
What factors are associated with a decrease in the rate and quality of the CRI?	1. Stress (mental, physical, emotional) 2. Chronic fatigue 3. Chronic infection 4. Depression 5. Other debilitating or psychiatric conditions	1.991, 10.177
Why can strains of the SBS be very significant?	Strains of the SBS can compromise the efficiency of the PRM, leading to dysfunction and disease.	1.992

What types of strains occur at the SBS?

Six types:
1. Torsions
2. Sidebending and rotation
3. Flexion and extension
4. Vertical
5. Lateral
6. Compression

1.992–993, 10.177

Which type of strain occurs around an AP axis, with the sphenoid and structures of the anterior cranium rotated in one direction, while the occiput and posterior cranium are rotated in the opposite direction?

A torsion strain

1.992–993

How is a torsion strain named?

It is named for the greater wing of the sphenoid that is more superior.

1.992–993

A sidebending and rotation strain occurs about what types of axes?

Rotation occurs about the AP axis, and sidebending occurs about two parallel vertical axes.

1.992–993

During a sidebending and rotation strain, do the sphenoid and occiput rotate in the same direction or in opposite directions?

The sphenoid and occiput rotate in the same direction.

1.992–993

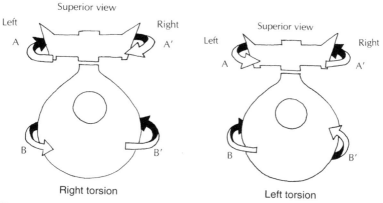

Figure 12–3.

How is a sidebending and rotation strain named?

This strain pattern is named for the side of convexity; the direction in which the sphenoid and occiput rotate when viewed from behind. Clockwise rotation would therefore be a right sidebending and rotation strain; conversely, counterclockwise rotation would be a left sidebending and rotation strain.

1.992–993

Which strain patterns are considered physiologic?

Torsion strains, in addition to sidebending and rotation strains, are considered physiologic because they do not interfere with the flexion or extension components of the PRM.

1.992–993, 10.176–177

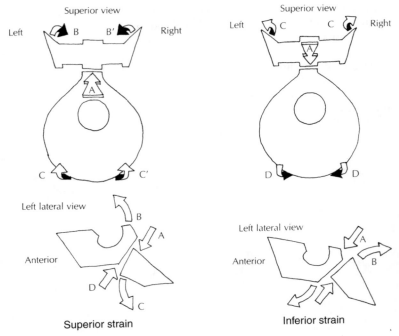

Figure 12–4.

When does a flexion and extension strain pattern occur?	It occurs when the motion at the SBS does not completely move through the flexion and extension phases equally and fully.	1.992–993
When is a vertical strain present?	When the sphenoid moves cephalad (superior vertical strain) or caudad (inferior vertical strain) in relation to the occiput around the two transverse axes	1.992–993
When is a lateral strain present?	When the sphenoid deviates laterally (left or right) in relation to the occiput around two parallel vertical axes	1.992–993
Which strain pattern is associated with a "parallelogram-shaped head", a strain that often occurs to infants in utero or during the birthing process?	A lateral strain	1.992–993

Superior view

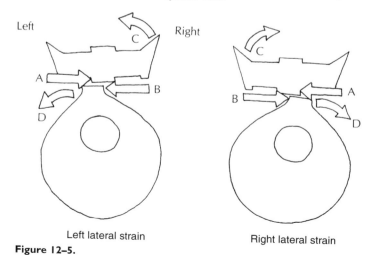

Left lateral strain

Right lateral strain

Figure 12–5.

Which strains may be superimposed on other strains?	Vertical and lateral strains	1.992–993
What is an SBS compression strain?	A strain where the occiput and sphenoid have been forced together, so that physiologic flexion and extension are impaired and even occasionally obliterated	10.181
Which strain pattern can significantly reduce the rate and amplitude of the CRI?	A compression strain	10.181
What type of situation can cause a compression strain?	Traumatic force to the back or front of the head, or circumferential compression of all sides of the head simultaneously, as in childbirth	1.993
Which bones are referred to as the paired bones of the skull?	The parietals, temporals, maxillae, zygoma, palatines, nasal, and frontal	10.171
Why is the frontal bone viewed as a paired bone?	Because the metopic suture (running down the center of the frontal bone) frequently remains open throughout life	10.171
What occurs during craniosacral flexion?	The SBS flexes, the foramen magnum elevates, and the base of the sacrum moves posterior (counternutates).	10.172
What occurs during craniosacral extension?	The SBS extends, the foramen magnum moves inferior, and the sacral base moves anterior (nutates).	10.172
What are the three layers of the dura?	1. Falx cerebri 2. Tentorium cerebelli 3. Falx cerebelli	10.176

What membrane separates the two cerebral hemispheres?	The falx cerebri	10.176
Which vascular structure does the falx cerebelli enclose?	The superior sagittal sinus	10.176
What dural layer separates the cerebrum and the cerebellum?	The tentorium cerebelli	10.176
Which vascular structure does the tentorium cerebelli enclose?	The transverse sinus	10.176
Where is the reciprocal tension (RTM) membrane located?	At the junction of the falx cerebri and tentorium cerebelli; the RTM is also sometimes referred to as the "Sutherland fulcrum."	10.176
What layer separates the two hemispheres of the cerebellum?	The falx cerebelli	10.176
How does respiration enhance SBS flexion and extension?	Inhalation enhances SBS flexion and exhalation enhances SBS extension.	10.177
Which dural layer is viewed as the "diaphragm" of the craniosacral mechanism?	The tentorium cerebelli	10.177
What happens to the tentorium cerebelli during inhalation?	The tentorium cerebelli descends and flattens during inhalation, as a result of external rotation of the temporal bones.	10.176–177
What happens to the tentorium cerebelli with SBS extension?	With SBS extension, enhanced by exhalation, the tentorium cerebelli elevates because of the internal rotation of the temporal bones	10.176–177

What hold technique is used to evaluate the SBS mechanics by placing the hands and fingers over the skull, and is also used as an indirect treatment to balance membranous tension?

The Vault hold technique

10.179

How are the physician's fingers placed when using the Vault hold?

1. Index fingers on the greater wing of the sphenoid
2. Pinky fingers on the occiput
3. The ear between the middle and ring fingers

10.179

What are the goals of the craniosacral techniques?

1. Balance the SBS motion
2. Reduce venous congestion
3. Enhance both the rate and amplitude of the CRI
4. Mobilize membranous articular restrictions and ultimately correct them

10.181–182

What is the primary activating force in craniosacral techniques?

Respiration (an inherent mechanism)

10.181–182

How is respiration used as an activating force?

Voluntary inhalation can enhance flexion of the midline bones and external rotation of the paired bones within the craniosacral mechanism.

10.183

Which type of lower extremity movement, dorsiflexion or plantarflexion, enhances flexion of the sphenobasilar junction?

Dorsiflexion

Note: Plantarflexion enhances extension of the SBS.

10.183

When using cranial techniques, what is a still point?

A sensation experienced where no motion is felt

10.183

What are the goals of the compression of the fourth ventricle (CV4) technique?	1. Enhance amplitude of the CRI 2. Enhance fluid movement 3. Restore function to the craniosacral mechanism	10.182–183
What is the goal of the venous sinus technique?	To enhance the flow of venous blood through venous sinuses	10.184
What technique is used to separate restricted and impacted sutures?	The V-spread technique	10.179–184
What are some of the complications associated with craniosacral treatments?	1. Alterations in heart rate, blood pressure, or respiration 2. gastrointestinal (GI) irritability 3. Tinnitus, dizziness, or headache	10.181–184
What are the contraindications to craniosacral treatment?	1. Acute intracranial bleeding or increased intracranial pressure 2. Skull trauma (fractures) 3. Seizures	10.179–184
Which cranial nerves (CN) are associated with suckling disorders and poor feeding in newborns?	CN IX, X, and XII are associated with occipital condylar compression, which can cause a poor feeding response in newborns.	1.1257, 1.667–674
Torticollis is associated with somatic dysfunction of which CN?	CN XI, because it supplies the sternocleidomastoid muscle, the muscle injured in torticollis	1.1257, 1.667–674
Dysfunction of the OA, AA, or C2 may affect the function of which CN?	CN X (vagus); dysfunction anywhere along the course of the vagus nerve can affect its normal function.	1.1257, 1.667–674
A lesion to which CN may cause arrythmias of the heart, difficulty coordinating digestion by the stomach and bowels, and trouble with breathing?	CN X (the vagus nerve)	13.351–353

Dysfunction affecting the jugular foramen can interfere with the normal function of which cranial nerves?	CN IX, X, and XI all pass through the jugular foramen.	1.1257, 1.667–674
Somatic dysfunction of which CN can be associated with vertigo or hearing loss?	CN VIII (the vestibulocochlear nerve)	1.1257, 1.667–674
Dysfunction of the ethmoid bone is associated with somatic dysfunction of which CN?	CN I (olfactory) dysfunction can produce an altered sense of smell.	1.1257, 1.667–674
Which CN exit the skull through the superior orbital fissure?	CN III (oculomotor), CN IV (trochlear), CN V (trigeminal) division 1, and CN VI (abducens)	13.346
CN XII exits the skull through which canal?	The hypoglossal canal	13.347
Injury to the cribiform plate of the ethmoid bone may cause anosmia by injuring which CN?	CN I (the olfactory nerve)	13.391
A lesion of which CN can cause bitemporal hemianopsia, better known as "tunnel vision"?	CN II (optic); this type of vision loss would occur with a lesion of CN II taking place at the optic chiasm.	13.391–392
A lesion to which CN will cause the ipsilateral eye to deviate downward and laterally, and ptosis?	CN III (oculomotor); the ptosis is caused by paralysis of the levator palpebrae superioris muscle.	13.392–393
A lesion of which CN as it exits the stylomastoid foramen can cause Bell's palsy?	CN VII (the facial nerve)	13.396

Which cranial nerve controls the afferent limb of the corneal blink reflex?	CN V (the trigeminal nerve) division 1, the ophthalmic division	13.394–395
Which division of the CN V (trigeminal) exits the skull through the foramen rotundum?	Division 2, the maxillary division	13.394–395
A narrowing of the foramen ovale would possibly compress what division of the trigeminal nerve?	Division 3, the mandibular division	13.394–395
A lesion to which CN would cause dysphagia and deviation of the tongue to the injured side?	CN XII (the hypoglossal nerve)	13.400
A lesion to which CN would eliminate the afferent limb of the gag reflex?	CN IX (the glossopharyngeal nerve)	13.398
A nerve lesion causing inflammation and swelling that compresses the dorsal aspect of the brainstem would most likely result in injury to which CN?	CN IV (trochlear), because it is the only CN to emerge from the dorsal aspect of the brainstem; it is also the smallest CN!	13.394

Chapter 13

Chapman Reflexes

What is the name for a viscerosomatic reflex mechanism that has diagnostic and therapeutic importance?	Chapman reflexes (points)	1.1051
What type of reflex is described as a neurolymphatic gangliform contraction that blocks lymphatic drainage, causing inflammation in tissues distal to the blockage, and causes both visceral and somatic tissues to suffer?	Chapman reflexes	1.1051
Today anterior Chapman points are most often used for what purpose?	To identify which organ is most likely dysfunctional	1.1051
Where are posterior Chapman reflexes usually located?	In the paraspinal area, near transverse processes	1.1051
On palpation, where are Chapman reflexes located?	Deep to the skin and subcutaneous areolar tissue, most often on the deep fascia or periosteum	1.1051
True or False: Chapman reflexes are usually found unpaired.	**False;** Chapman reflexes are usually found paired on both the ventral and dorsal surfaces of the body.	1.1051
True or False: Compression of an anterior Chapman point reveals a firm, painless mass.	**False;** Chapman reflexes cause greater pain than expected by both the patient and physician, even with light compression.	1.1051

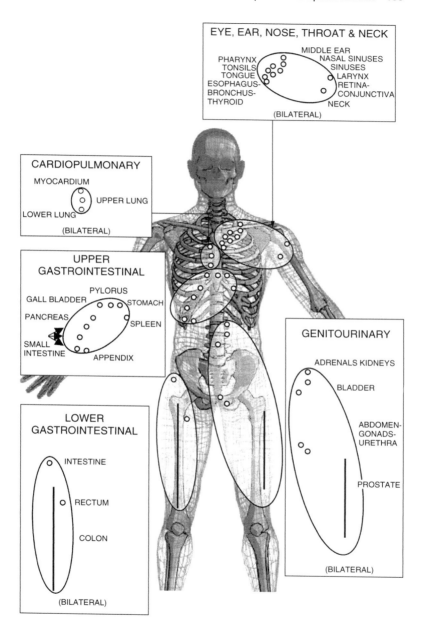

EYE, EAR, NOSE, THROAT & NECK

MIDDLE EAR
PHARYNX
TONSILS
TONGUE
ESOPHAGUS-
BRONCHUS-
THYROID
NASAL SINUSES
SINUSES
LARYNX
RETINA-
CONJUNCTIVA
NECK
(BILATERAL)

CARDIOPULMONARY

MYOCARDIUM
UPPER LUNG
LOWER LUNG
(BILATERAL)

UPPER
GASTROINTESTINAL

PYLORUS
GALL BLADDER
STOMACH
PANCREAS
SPLEEN
SMALL
INTESTINE
APPENDIX

GENITOURINARY

ADRENALS KIDNEYS
BLADDER
ABDOMEN-
GONADS-
URETHRA
PROSTATE
(BILATERAL)

LOWER
GASTROINTESTINAL

INTESTINE
RECTUM
COLON
(BILATERAL)

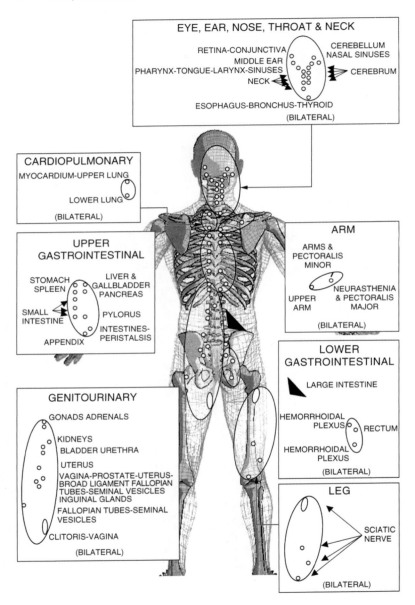

EYE, EAR, NOSE, THROAT & NECK

RETINA-CONJUNCTIVA
MIDDLE EAR
PHARYNX-TONGUE-LARYNX-SINUSES
NECK

CEREBELLUM
NASAL SINUSES
CEREBRUM

ESOPHAGUS-BRONCHUS-THYROID
(BILATERAL)

CARDIOPULMONARY
MYOCARDIUM-UPPER LUNG

LOWER LUNG
(BILATERAL)

UPPER GASTROINTESTINAL

STOMACH
SPLEEN

LIVER &
GALLBLADDER
PANCREAS

SMALL
INTESTINE

PYLORUS

APPENDIX

INTESTINES-
PERISTALSIS

ARM

ARMS &
PECTORALIS
MINOR

UPPER
ARM

NEURASTHENIA
& PECTORALIS
MAJOR

(BILATERAL)

LOWER GASTROINTESTINAL

LARGE INTESTINE

HEMORRHOIDAL
PLEXUS

RECTUM

HEMORRHOIDAL
PLEXUS

(BILATERAL)

GENITOURINARY

GONADS ADRENALS

KIDNEYS
BLADDER URETHRA

UTERUS
VAGINA-PROSTATE-UTERUS-
BROAD LIGAMENT FALLOPIAN
TUBES-SEMINAL VESICLES
INGUINAL GLANDS
FALLOPIAN TUBES-SEMINAL
VESICLES

CLITORIS-VAGINA

(BILATERAL)

LEG

SCIATIC
NERVE

(BILATERAL)

What are five distinguishing characteristics of Chapman reflexes?

Nodules that are
1. Small
2. Smooth
3. Firm
4. Discretely palpable (or grouped in irregular patches)
5. About 2 to 3 mm in diameter when palpated alone

1.1051

To an examining physician, how do Chapman reflexes feel?

1. Like small pearls of tapioca lying partially fixed on the deep fascia
2. Dense but not hard
3. Circumscribed area of firm edema
4. Fixed (cannot be displaced)

1.1051

Are confluent areas of Chapman reflexes acute or chronic?

Chronic; confluent (flowing and blended into one) reflexes, although rare, are thought to represent longstanding visceral reflexes of greater magnitude and chronicity than single discrete masses.

1.1051

How is the pain from compression of a Chapman reflex characteristically described?

1. Nonradiating
2. Exquisitely distressing
3. Sharp
4. Pinpoint
5. Painful ganglioform contractions

1.1052

True or False: Patients usually do not realize they have Chapman reflexes present.

True; patients usually grimace and withdraw from the pain caused by light compression of a Chapman reflex but experience only mild symptoms with much deeper pressure.

1.1052

Where is the Chapman reflex located for patients suffering from acute appendicitis?

At the tip of the right twelfth rib. This a commonly tested question on the board examination.

1.1052

Frank Chapman, believing in the interconnectedness and interrelatedness of the body as described by A.T. Still's four basic osteopathic principles, suggested treatment of what area before addressing Chapman reflexes?

Chapman suggested that treatment of a pelvic dysfunction initially noticeably enhanced the response to subsequent treatment of Chapman reflexes.

1.1052

How are Chapman reflexes of the colon located and correlated?

By flipping the colon 180° upon a transverse axis through the cecum and low sigmoid regions, so that the right proximal colon lies on the right femoral head, the right ascending colon runs along the anterior aspect of the femur, and the hepatic flexure lies just superior to the patella (with the same relationship for the descending colon upon the left femur)

1.1053

A Chapman reflex located on the trochanter of the right hip is associated with dysfunction of what structure?

The cecum

1.1053

A Chapman reflex located on the distal portion of the left femur is associated with dysfunction of what structure?

The splenic flexure

1.1053

A Chapman reflex located on the proximal portion of the left femur is associated with dysfunction of what structure?

The sigmoid colon and rectum

1.1053

An anterior Chapman reflex located just laterally to the superior surface of the pubic symphysis is associated with dysfunction of what structures?

Ovaries and urethra

1.1053

The anterior Chapman reflex for cerebellar problems is located where?	The coracoid process	1.1053
The anterior Chapman reflex for the liver only is located where?	In the right intercostal space between ribs 5 and 6	1.1052
The anterior Chapman reflex for the liver and gallbladder is located where?	In the right intercostal space between the ribs 6 and 7	1.1052
The anterior Chapman reflex for the pylorus and its sphincter is located where?	On the anterior surface of the sternum	1.1052
The anterior Chapman reflex for stomach acidity is located where?	In the left intercostal space between ribs 5 and 6	1.1052
The anterior Chapman reflex for stomach peristalsis is located where?	In the left intercostal space between ribs 6 and 7	1.1052
The anterior Chapman reflex for intestinal peristalsis is located where?	Below the inguinal ligament, just lateral to the anterior inferior iliac spine (AIIS)	1.1053
The anterior Chapman reflex for the prostate and broad ligament is located where?	On the lateral aspect of the femur	1.1053
Thyroid problems can cause an anterior Chapman reflex located where?	In the intercostal space between ribs 2 and 3	1.1053
Somatic dysfunction of what structures, other than the thyroid, can cause anterior Chapman points in the intercostal space between the second and third rib?	Bronchus, esophagus, and myocardium	1.1053

An anterior Chapman reflex located on the inferior pubic ramus is associated with dysfunction of what structure?	The uterus	1.1053
An anterior Chapman reflex located on the humerus, just superior to the deltoid tuberosity, is associated with dysfunction of what structures?	The retina and conjuctiva	1.1053
What anterior Chapman reflexes are located in the intercostal space between ribs 1 and 2?	1. Nasal sinuses 2. Pharynx 3. Tonsils 4. Tongue 5. Larynx 6. Sinuses	1.1053
Anterior Chapman reflexes located in the intercostal spaces between ribs 8 and 9, ribs 9 and 10, and ribs 10 and 11 is associated with dysfunction of what structure?	The small intestines	1.1053
An anterior Chapman reflex located in the intercostal space between the third and fourth ribs is associated with dysfunction of what structure?	The upper lung	1.1053
An anterior Chapman reflex located in the intercostal space between the fourth and fifth ribs is associated with dysfunction of what structure?	The lower lung	1.1053
An anterior Chapman reflex located 1 inch laterally and 2 inches superiorly to the umbilicus is associated with dysfunction of what structure?	The adrenals	1.1053

An anterior Chapman reflex located 1 inch laterally and 1 inch superiorly to the umbilicus is associated with dysfunction of what structure?	The kidneys	1.1053
An anterior Chapman reflex located periumbilically is associated with dysfunction of what structure?	The bladder	1.1053
An anterior Chapman reflex located in the left intercostal space between the ribs 7 and 8 is associated with dysfunction of what structure?	The spleen	1.1053
An anterior Chapman reflex located in the right intercostal space between ribs 7 and 8 is associated with dysfunction of what structure?	The pancreas	1.1053
A posterior Chapman reflex located near the transverse process of the eleventh thoracic vertebra is associated with dysfunction of what structure and known to be found in some hypertensive patients?	The adrenals	1.1054
How are Chapman points treated?	1. Initially, pelvic function must be normalized. 2. Apply heavy (even uncomfortable) pressure to the gangliform mass. 3. Use slow, circular movements with the finger in an effort to flatten out the mass as if it were a localized fluid accumulation. 4. Continue to perform the moving pressure for 10 to 30 seconds.	1.1055

5. Cease treatment when the mass disappears or the treatment can no longer be tolerated.

Treatment of what posterior Chapman reflexes aid in decreasing blood pressure in hypertensive patients?

The adrenal Chapman points; decreased blood pressure, as well as decreased serum aldosterone levels, are seen as soon as 36 hours after the soft tissue treatment.

1.1055

True or False: Chapman reflexes are highly efficient diagnostic tools, even among more expensive diagnostic tools.

This is accepted as true within the osteopathic research and literature.

1.1055

Chapter 14

Travell Trigger Points

What is a myofascial trigger point (TP)?	A hyperirritable spot in skeletal muscles associated with a hypersensitive palpable nodule in a taut band; it is painful upon compression and can give rise to a characteristic referred pain, referred tenderness, motor dysfunction, and autonomic phenomena.	1.1035–1037
Do TPs refer pain?	**Yes;** in fact, the term TP is reserved for **only** those myofascial points that have the potential to refer pain.	1.1037
Do TPs refer pain in any direction?	**No,** TPs are known to refer pain in a certain predictable distribution.	1.1037
What are the two types of TPs, based on their ability to refer pain?	Active and latent TPs	1.1037
What is an active TP?	A TP that refers pain at rest, with muscular activity, or with palpation	1.1037
What type of TP refers pain only when probed with a very steady pressure?	Latent TPs	1.1037
Which type of TPs are often overlooked or misdiagnosed by novice palpatory examiners because they are difficult to identify?	Latent TPs	1.1037

To where does the pain from a TP in the deep portion of the masseter muscle radiate most strongly?	The external auditory ear canal and into the middle ear; less radiating pain is felt on the lateral portion of the face surrounding the muscle.	1.1035
Which TP is compressed if a patient experiences radiating pain that migrates from the ipsilateral side of the face above the eye across to the above the eye?	The clavicular portion of the sternocleidomastoid TP	1.1035
What TP radiates pain over the entire "big" toe?	The tibialis anterior TP	1.1036
In which muscle are TPs most likely to develop?	The upper trapezius muscle	1.1038
What diseases and (or) conditions seem to perpetuate TPs?	1. Chronic infections 2. Allergic rhinitis 3. Psychological stressors 4. Endocrine and metabolic disorders, including hypothyroidism and hypoglycemia	1.1038
What is one of the strongest factors contributing to the formation and perpetuation of TPs?	Overuse of somatic structures, especially chilled muscles (caused by an improper warm-up period before physical exertion or an improper cool down after a workout followed by a strenuous movement)	1.1038
Which two physicians are credited with bringing TPs into the public eye?	Travell and Simon; much of their public notoriety came from treating President John F. Kennedy.	1.1038

The tenderness and pain associated with TPs are due to what chemical mediators?	Prostaglandins, potassium, substance P, bradykinins, serotonin, histamine, and leukotrienes	1.1038
What manifests itself as a nodular or spindle-shaped thickening of the tissues with alterations in cutaneous temperature and humidity?	A myofascial (Travell) TP	1.1038
What is a "jump sign"?	Wincing or withdrawal of the patient due to pain and discomfort, seen with a resultant "local twitch" of a taut muscle band when compressed	1.1038
What causes a "jump sign"?	A myofascial (Travell) TP	1.1038
What kinds of mechanical abuse can lead to the formation of a TP?	1. Muscle overload 2. Myofascial postural stress 3. Leaving a muscle in a prolonged shortened position, especially if the muscle is then quickly contracted from that position 4. Muscle chilling	1.1039
Successful treatment of myofascial TPs depends on what four elements?	Removing the primary myofascial TP, its associated satellite TPs, related articular dysfunction, and any underlying or perpetuating factors	1.1039
The local twitch response usually helps differentiate which musculoskeletal disorders?	The local twitch response, a transient contraction of the taut band of fibers housing a TP, is usually absent in fibromyalgia but present in myofascial pain syndromes caused by TPs.	1.1039

What factors ensure that treatment of a TP will last?

1. Correction of the associated somatic dysfunction
2. Educating patient to prevent recurrences
3. Appropriate self-stretch exercise programs
4. Correction of underlying perpetual and facilitating factors

1.1040

What specific techniques have been used to treat myofascial TPs?

1. Inhibition soft tissue techniques
2. Vasocoolant spray or other intermittent cooling measures with stretch
3. Deep massage
4. Injection
5. Jones counterstrain
6. Isometric muscle energy techniques
7. Myofascial release

1.1040–1041

Works Cited

1. Ward RC, ed. Foundations for Osteopathic Medicine. 2nd ed. Philadelphia: Lippincott Williams & Wilkins, 2003.

2. Speece CA, Crow WT. Ligamentous Articular Strain: Osteopathic Manipulative Techniques for the Body. Seattle, WA: Eastland Press, 2001.

3. Kuchera WA, Kuchera ML, eds. Osteopathic Principles in Practice. 2nd rev, ed. Columbus, OH: Greyden Press, 1993.

4. Kimberly PE. Outline of Osteopathic Manipulative Procedure: The Kimberly Manual, Millennium Edition. Kimberly PE, Funk SL, eds. Kirksville, MO: Kirksville College of Osteopathic Medicine, 2000.

5. Moore KL, Agur AMR. Essential Clinical Anatomy. 2nd ed. Baltimore: Lippincott Williams & Wilkins, 2002.

6. DiGiovanna EL, Schiowitz S, Dowling DJ, eds. An Osteopathic Approach to Diagnosis and Treatment. 3rd ed. Philadelphia: Lippincott Williams & Wilkins, 2005.

7. Snell RS. Clinical Anatomy. 7th ed. Baltimore: Lippincott Williams & Wilkins, 2004.

8. Hansen JT, Lambert DR, eds. Netter's Clinical Anatomy. Carlstadt, NJ: Icon Learning Systems, Novartis Medical Education, 2005.

9. Moore KL, Dalley AF. Clinically Oriented Anatomy. 5th ed. Baltimore: Lippincott Williams & Wilkins, 2006.

10. Greenman PE. Principles of Manual Medicine. 3rd ed. Philadelphia: Lippincott Williams & Wilkins, 2003.

11. Jones LH, Kusunose R, Goering E. Jones Strain-CounterStrain. American Academy of Osteopathy. Boise, ID: Jones Strain-CounterStrain, Inc., 1995.

12. DiGiovanna EL, Schiowitz S. An Osteopathic Approach to Diagnosis and Treatment. 2nd ed. Philadelphia: Lippincott, 1997.

13. Chung KW. BRS Gross Anatomy. 5th ed. Baltimore: Lippincott Williams & Wilkins, 2005.

Figure Credits

Figures 1-1, 2-2, 2-5, and all figures in Chapters 12 and 13:

DiGiovanna EL, Schiowitz S, Dowling DJ, eds. An Osteopathic Approach to Diagnosis and Treatment. 3rd ed. Philadelphia: Lippincott Williams & Wilkins, 2005.

Figures 2-1 and all figures in Chapter 7:

Modi RG, Shah NA. COMLEX Review: Clinical Anatomy and Osteopathic Manipulative Medicine. Malden, MA: Blackwell Publishing, 2006.

Figure 2-3:

Ward RC, ed. Foundations for Osteopathic Medicine. 2nd ed. Philadelphia: Lippincott Williams & Wilkins, 2003.

Index

Page numbers followed by *f* or *t* indicate figures or tables, respectively.

OSTEOPATHIC MEDICINE RECALL

RECALL SERIES EDITOR

LORNE H. BLACKBOURNE, MD
Trauma, Burn, and Critical Care Surgeon
San Antonio, Texas